The Complete

Tai Chi Tutor

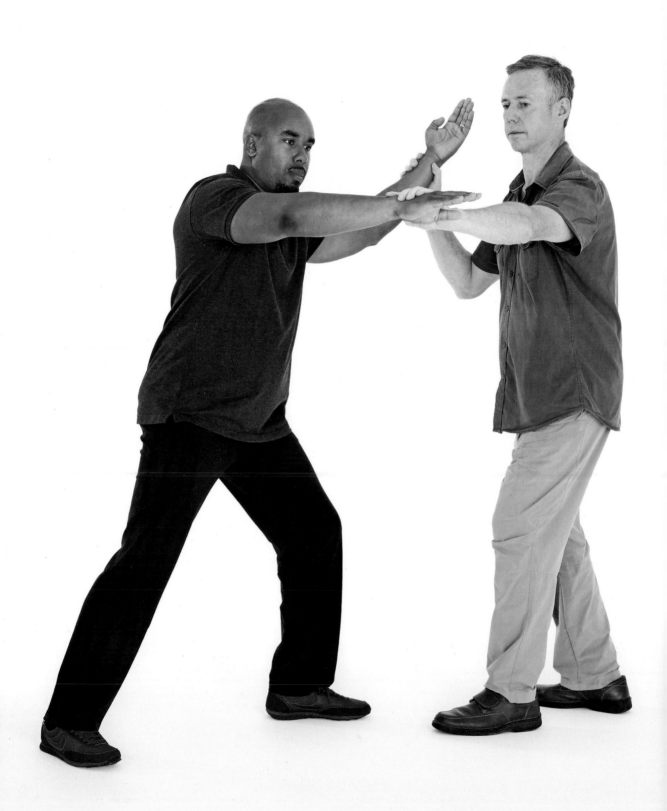

The Complete
Tai Chi
Tutor

A structured course to achieve
professional expertise

Dan Docherty

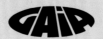

In memoriam:

Inspector Charles Edward Docherty

(1960–2013)

An Hachette UK Company
www.hachette.co.uk

First published in Great Britain
in 2015 by Gaia, a division of
Octopus Publishing Group Ltd
Carmelite House,
50 Victoria Embankment
London EC4Y 0DZ
www.octopusbooks.co.uk

ISBN 978-1-85675-352-4

A CIP catalogue record for this book is
available from the British Library

Printed and bound in China

10 9 8 7 6 5 4 3 2 1

All reasonable care has been taken in the
preparation of this book, but the information
it contains is not meant to take the place of
medical care under the direct supervision
of a doctor. Before making any changes in
your health regime, always consult a doctor.
While all the practices detailed in this book
are completely safe if done correctly, you
must seek professional advice if you are in
any doubt about any medical condition. Any
application of the ideas and information
contained in this book is at the reader's sole
discretion and risk.

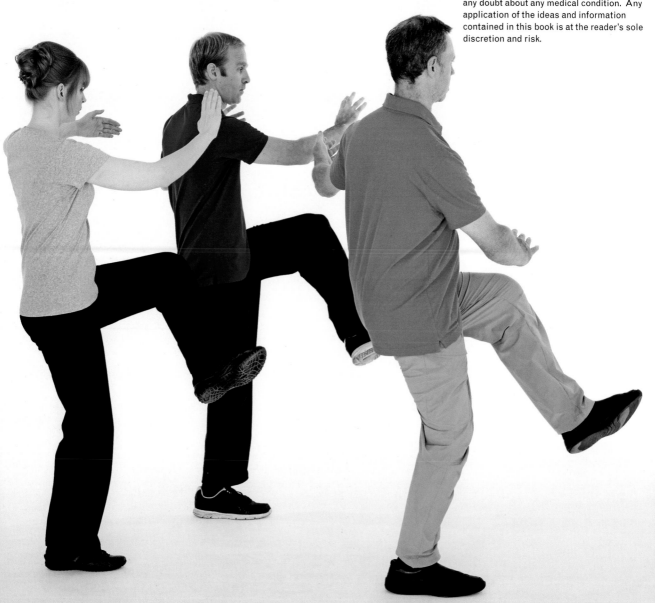

Contents

Introduction

'Some are born with knowledge, some get it by study, some obtain the knowledge after painfully sensing their ignorance.'

'To be fond of learning is to be near to knowledge.'

THE DOCTRINE OF THE MEAN

This book is a personal tuition book for those who wish to learn Tai Chi, for those who wish to teach Tai Chi and for those who are already teaching Tai Chi, but want to become more skilled in their practice, in their knowledge of Tai Chi history and theory, and in their instruction. Not only is the book complete in terms of its target audience, it is also complete in that it covers all aspects of Tai Chi history, theory and practice, including lost traditions. The practical sections of the book include detailed analysis of key techniques and partner work.

In a sense it's easy to learn Tai Chi – badly. Many practitioners are able to do only some basic movements. This book is here to teach you that Tai Chi can be a whole lot more interesting and fun for tutor and student on both a physical and an intellectual level.

Different readers will assimilate the information contained herein at different speeds. That's okay. It's not a race.

A tutor is a teacher and a bit more than that. In Roman law a tutor was an adult who looked after the interests of a child under the age of puberty. Nowadays the term suggests a private teacher/instructor/mentor who has some degree of personal involvement in the life of those under his charge. This is very much what is meant by the Cantonese term Sifu, used in Kung Fu movies as a term of respect for a Kung Fu master, but also applied (outside the movie world) to a Tai Chi tutor. Shifu is Mandarin dialect for the same two characters, but I'll use the Cantonese version as it is better known.

The character for Si/Shi means commander/master/mastery. Fu can be one of two different characters, one of which means father, the other a tutor/instructor. Sifu are indeed considered to be fathers of their martial arts family, though the term is not restricted to martial arts. Laoshi, meaning old/revered teacher, is also sometimes used, as is the modern mainland Chinese term Jiaolian, coach/trainer. Students of martial arts are referred to as Tudi, which literally means 'apprentice younger brother' – that is, disciple. Once they have undergone the Baishi/Respect the Master ceremony, they become Men Ren, 'inside the door students'.

Chinese society, Chinese martial arts and Tai Chi schools are all hierarchical in nature. Students are regarded as each other's 'older' and 'younger' brothers and sisters, mainly on the basis of when they started training in their school, but sometimes according to age and ability. In my teacher's school in Hong Kong, for example, my old training partner Tong Chi-kin and I were addressed by many older students as 'big elder brother' as we were South-East Asian Chinese full-contact champions.

Over the years I've tutored many students needing special attention: some because of health problems, some because of bullying, some because they were particularly talented in the sports/competition aspect of Tai Chi and required more advanced material. This last type of student is often exceptionally capable and highly motivated. I also have taught hundreds of people how to teach Tai Chi and how to be better Tai Chi teachers – complete Tai Chi tutors.

Author's note

For ease of reference, I have used mainly the modern Chinese romanization system known as pinyin, which comes from mainland China and is based on the standard Mandarin dialect.

Please consult the Glossary on page 230 for an explanation of any unfamiliar terms mentioned in the text.

Being a Tai Chi Tutor

Tai Chi tutoring is important on a cultural level too. I actively encourage students to learn Chinese and to visit the Far East. From 1975–84 I lived in Hong Kong, serving as a Senior Inspector in the Royal Hong Kong Police Force and successfully representing Hong Kong in Chinese International full-contact fighting, using Tai Chi to defeat fighters from a hard-style Kung Fu background.

Before that I had trained in Karate in Glasgow, Scotland, for four years and in 1974 was awarded a black belt. I'd read about Tai Chi and was very interested, but couldn't understand how it worked from the books then available. I took it up seriously in Hong Kong in 1975 with a teacher named Cheng Tin-hung, who had taught a lot of international Chinese full-contact fighters – and a lot of police officers. Within five minutes of meeting him I was convinced that Sifu Cheng was the tutor for me. I never regretted that decision. He was fast, focused, skilful and fat.

Since 1984, I've visited all the important sites associated with Chinese martial arts: I've taken groups of Tai Chi students and friends up, down and around the Wudang Mountains 12 times. I've been to the Northern Shaolin Temple five times and once, on the back of a motorbike, to the Southern Shaolin Temple in Quanzhou. I've been to all the famous and some not-so-famous Tai Chi places: the Forbidden City, the White Cloud Temple, Baoji, the Huashan, Hengshan (Hua and Heng Mountains), Chenjiagou (the Chen family village), Zhaobao, Shanghai and Guangping. I've read all I could find on Chinese culture and martial arts. I've taken students to compete in France, Holland, Russia, Denmark, Sweden, the USA, Taiwan, Hong Kong and China.

This book is the distilled essence of those experiences, fights and pilgrimages. This book is your complete Tai Chi tutor. We'll investigate what is known and unknown concerning the origins and history of Tai Chi, following its tracks through the most ancient texts of Chinese civilization to the 21st century and trying to resolve some key questions on the way. We'll consider the practicalities of teaching, reviewing the fundamentals and benefits of practise, and we'll learn some highly efficacious but little known drills. Finally, we look into the nature of Tai Chi expertise and explore areas of specialist interest, in terms of tuition and styles, as well as studies and writings on Tai Chi.

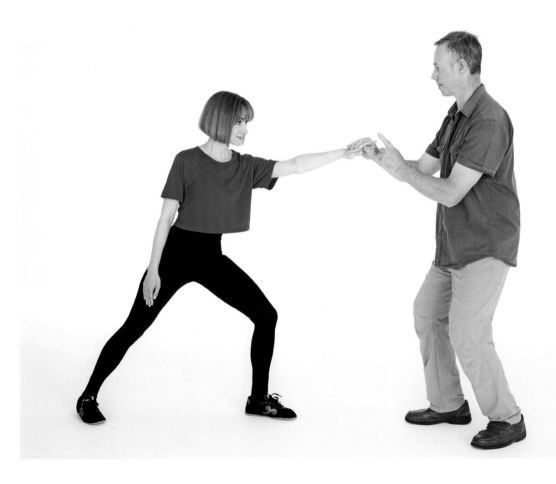

Getting Started

Learning Tai Chi

The first thing is to try to find a tutor who is ready, willing and able to teach you the type of Tai Chi that you want to learn. The coming of the internet has made this process a lot easier, but nothing beats personal contact. If possible go and see a few different teachers so you can compare approaches and see what suits you. The tutor may be highly skilled, but you need to look at what his students can do, as potentially you're going to be one of them.

Everybody told me not to give up my legal career in order to go out and join the Royal Hong Kong Police Force (which I thought would be the most practical way to get to the Far East to learn Tai Chi properly). I didn't listen. I did it anyway.

Teaching Tai Chi

Some people just want the kudos of being a Tai Chi Sifu. Some want to have people to train with. Some want a change of career. Whatever the reason, becoming a Tai Chi tutor requires a considerable commitment in terms of time, energy and money (I know some teachers who run classes at a loss).

Everybody told me not to give up my police career to move to London and become a Tai Chi tutor from scratch. I didn't listen. I did it anyway.

In the words of the philosopher Laozi, 'A journey of a thousand Li (Chinese kilometres) begins at your feet.'

Let's start the journey.

Understanding Tai Chi

Most of the key concepts of Tai Chi are found in a body of work known collectively as the five Tai Chi Chuan Classics: most of them were first written down in the 19th century, but contain oral traditions that have been passed down through many generations.

The individual titles are *The Canon of Tai Chi Chuan*, *The Fighter's Song*, *An Interpretation of the Practice of the 13 Tactics*, *The Song of the 13 Tactics* and *The Tai Chi Chuan Discourse*. In order to get the most out of our Tai Chi practice, we need to understand certain basic things that the Classics tell us and we shall refer to them as necessary throughout the book.

The Tai Chi Chuan Discourse begins, 'When you move, the whole body must be light and agile. In particular it must be linked together.'

This means we need to have good posture, which is achieved by maintaining a more or less straight line from the crown of the head through to the tailbone, though the angle of this line changes according to our movements. When we move, everything is connected, everything starts and finishes together.

We need also to train footwork and weight transference; the basic Seven Star Step drill is highly effective in delivering these qualities. It's the first thing I teach to beginners. In the drill we link the body by coordinating zigzag forward stepping with pushes, then stepping back in a zigzag and diverting to the side with our arms. A detailed explanation of the drill is given in my book *The Tai Chi Bible*.

The Tai Chi Chuan Discourse continues, 'The root is in the feet. Discharging is done by the legs. The controlling power is in the waist and the appearance is in the hands and fingers.'

For example, the Tai Chi Sabre Form contains a lot of sequences of crouching like a tiger and then lunging forward as a tiger does to seize its prey. When we crouch, our centre of gravity is low and the feet are as if rooted to the ground. The lunge is the discharge of force and is performed by suddenly thrusting forward, straightening the rear leg and stepping forward with the front foot.

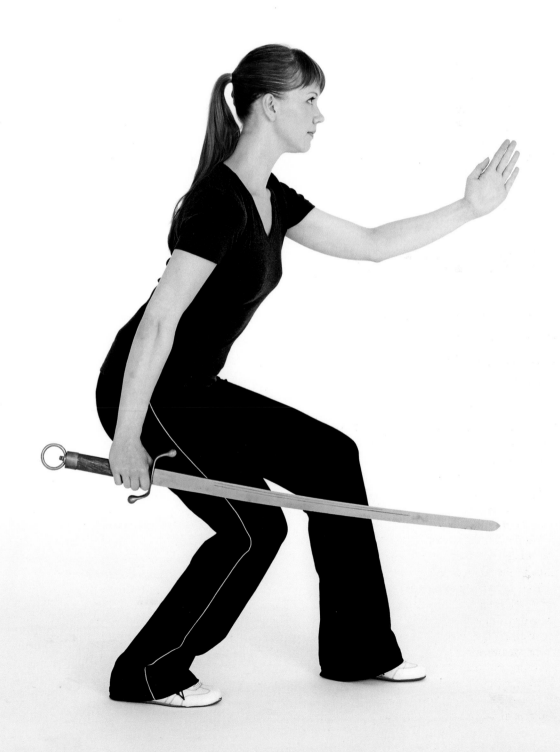

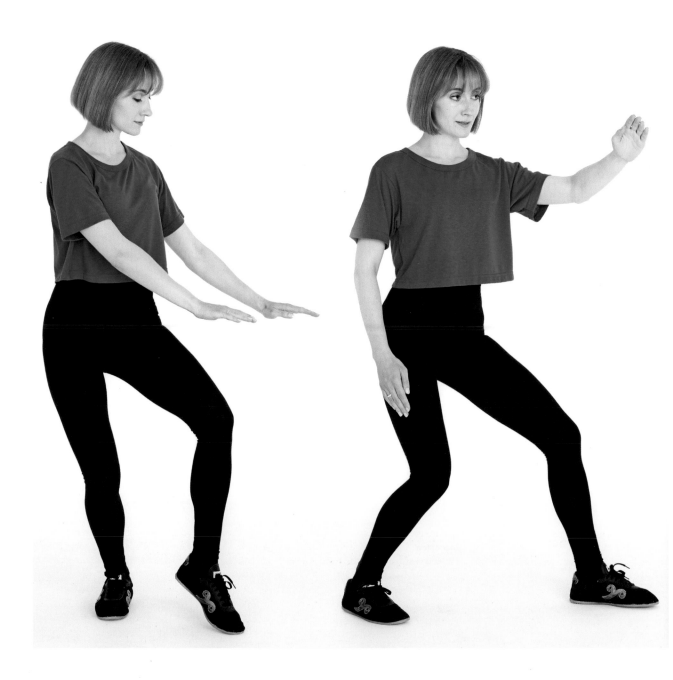

Above The knees are bent to lower the centre of gravity and so become rooted.

'Rooting' is a key Tai Chi skill. In order to 'root', our stances need to be deep, so that the centre of gravity is lowered. This in turn helps us to generate more thrust from the legs. It isn't really the waist that controls things, it's the rotation of the spinal column as, for example, in the Seven Star Step, when we step forward to push and step back to divert. To the beginner it looks as if we are just moving the hands and fingers.

'From the feet to the legs to the waist, all must be completely uniform and done in one breath.'

The Canon of Tai Chi Chuan connects Tai Chi Chuan with Chinese philosophy, but is mainly concerned with using duality (as in the concept of Yin and Yang) and change, distance and timing, in order to understand and use educated force (Jin) to deal with an opponent's attacks in a harmonious way. At the same time we follow the Taoist principle of oneness. Yin and Yang are not separate, but together make a whole thing that we call Tai Chi. The Sabre Form crouch and thrust is a whole thing. Making it so requires Pushing Hands and application training (in Tai Chi, Pushing Hands is a technical term meaning to feel or sense what the opponent is doing. Application training is the practice of individual Tai Chi self-defence techniques against one or more opponents. Most, but not all of these techniques, can be found in the Tai Chi Hand Form, though in some cases the practical application of a technique may be rather different from the way it is executed in the hand form.).

An Interpretation of the Practice of the 13 Tactics is mainly concerned with the cultivation and circulation of Qi/vital energy and the respective roles of Xin/the heart mind and Shen/the Spirit.

'Xin is the commander...the Shen is at ease and the body is tranquil.'

This Classic also discusses Jin/educated force in action:

'By using the curve to gather the Jin, there is more than a sufficiency.'

The Song of the 13 Tactics mentions Kung Fu, in the sense of effort, three times. It also emphasizes the use of intent and the mind, as well as the importance of correct posture in Qi circulation.

'Every tactic lives in the Xin; the principle is to use the Yi/intent.'

'Kung Fu is unceasing.'

The Fighter's Song deals with strategy and the use of force, advising us to be ready to follow up our initial technique and expect the opponent to do likewise.

'The technique is broken, but the intent is unbroken.'

A complete translation of all five Tai Chi Chuan Classics, with an illustrated commentary, is to be found in my book Tai Chi Chuan – Decoding the Classics for the Modern Martial Artist.

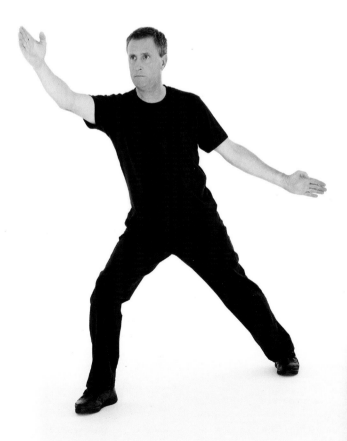

Right Using the curve to gather the Jin.

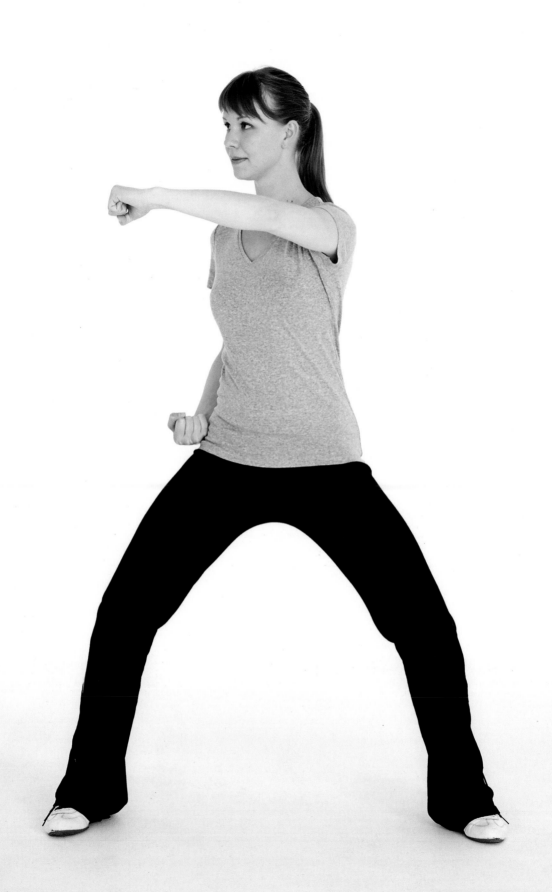

1 The Lost Tai Chi

Tai Chi is a huge and complex jigsaw, and quite a few pieces seem to be missing or belong to another puzzle entirely. In this section, we'll re-examine some old and, to some readers, familiar Chinese texts – what we can call 'known knowns'. We will then look at sources that are vaguely known to be important in the development of Tai Chi (though this connexion is not at all understood) – the 'known unknowns'. Finally, we'll explore more esoteric and recondite material which the average reader may be unaware of – the 'unknown unknowns'. Along the way we'll no doubt meet some 'unknown knowns': things that we think we know, but which we really don't know.

All classical Chinese texts are full of accretions, revisions, borrowings, interpolations and extrapolations. There are no exceptions among those we are about to examine. I refer in this chapter to chanting/reciting from The Tai Chi Chuan Classics, and in fact, classical Chinese writings were largely memorized in this way.

The historical origins of and cultural influences on the art of Tai Chi are not well understood, except by a few diehards. My hope is to reclaim at least some of this lost Tai Chi and to help recreate the puzzle.

As always with Tai Chi, it's the journey which is important.

The Known Tai Chi

In this chapter, we'll attempt to trace how elements of divination, poetry, philosophy and military strategy combined with Chinese medicine and holistic exercise and with Chinese martial arts through the ages to produce the art we now call Tai Chi Chuan – the philosophical concept of Tai Chi expressed in a sophisticated martial art. Some of these influences such as *The Book of Changes* and the philosophy of Laozi will be familiar, though I'm sure many readers will find some interesting personal unknowns in these famous texts, too. Texts such as Nei Ye/Inward Training are more obscure and clearly part of a 'lost' Tai Chi.

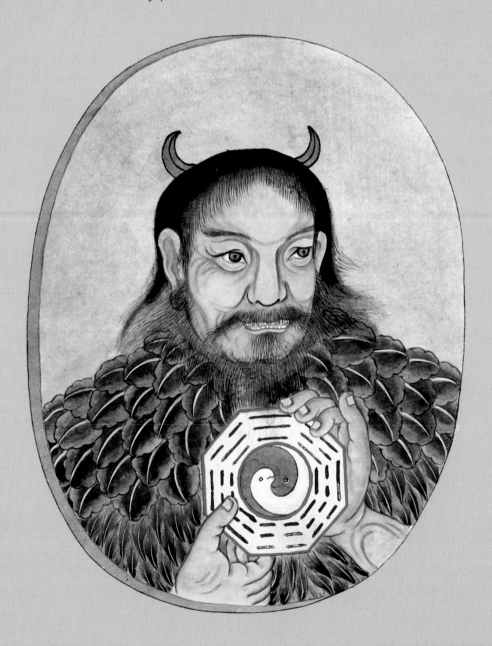

The Beginning – Chinese Cosmology

Before analysing the Tai Chi symbol and Yin/Yang theory, it is helpful to examine the basic Chinese concepts of the universe. Traced from about 1000 BCE and developed by succeeding philosophers and schools of philosophy, they are as follows:

Tao (Way) cannot be spoken of and has no name (Laozi Chapter 1). In other words it is …

↓

Wu (Nothing) According to Laozi (Chapter 2), something and nothing mutually gave birth to one another, so we have Wu Chi yet Tai Chi; Wu Wei (not to act against Nature) is Tao and from it came …

↓

Hun Tun (Chaos), which is also Tai Chi (Supreme Ultimate/Pole), a potentiality containing form, Qi (energy/vapour) and substance.

↓

Tai Yi (Supreme Change) took place and produced …

↓

Tai Chu (Supreme Starting) of form and shape which caused …

↓

Tai Shi (Supreme Beginning) of Qi and then …

↓

Tai Xu (Supreme Emptiness), which brought the formation of substance and was the origin of…

↓

Liang Yi (Two Principles) known as **Yin (passive, female)** and **Yang (active, male)**, the interaction of which produced…

Wu Xing (Five Elements) of Fire, Water, Wood, Earth and Metal, which in turn produced…

↓

The Ten Thousand Things, including… Humanity, which is composed of Yin and Yang.

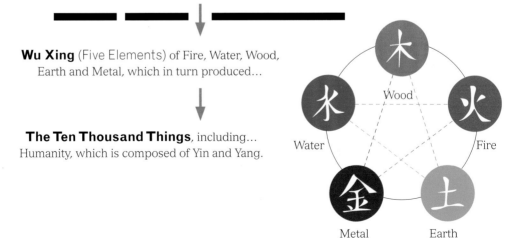

Wood

Water

Fire

Metal

Earth

In Taoist lore, Yin governs the seven emotions, which on death descend to earth to become Gui or demon; Yang governs the internal alchemy of Qi, Jing and Shen, which on death ascend to heaven to become a spirit or immortal.

Much of the theory and terminology of Tai Chi Chuan is derived from these concepts and those who developed the art would have been well versed in them. The original symbol for the concept of Tai Chi seems to have been a simple circle. This is logical, as once we have a circle there is an inside and an outside, what is enclosed and what is not, what is circular and what is not – we have Yin and Yang. The inspiration for the circle may have come from the sun or moon. Over the years the black and white symbol for Liang Yi/Two Principles – that is, Yin and Yang – replaced the simple circle and became known as the Tai Chi symbol.

Taoism

This important Chinese religion had two origins. The first was with the philosophers of the Warring States Period (475–221 BCE), who followed the way of harmony with nature. The second was among the shamans and magicians from China's northern periphery who attempted to intercede with gods and demons. These two threads later combined to form the Taoist religion.

The prolongation of life and hence cultivation of Yang energy has long been a major goal of Taoism. Connections between Tai Chi and Taoism are therefore hardly surprising.

Laozi (c. 5th century BCE)

Tai Chi theory has often been linked by its many practitioners with the writings of the philosopher Laozi (literally Old Boy) and his book, *The Classic of the Way and Virtue*. My old friend and esteemed Tai Chi scholar Dr Marnix Wells once correctly pointed out that The Tai Chi Chuan Classics contain no direct quotes from Laozi, yet in Laozi's writings there are many references to duality similar in tone to those later found in The Tai Chi Chuan Classics. For example,

• 'Bowed down then whole, bent then straight, hollow then full' brings to mind Fuyang/Bow Down Look Up Pushing Hands.

• The line from *An Interpretation of the Practice of the 13 Tactics*, 'Seek the straight amid the bent', which can be a reference to straightening the joints without locking them out or to bending the limbs in defence and straightening them when countering (see below).

• *The Tai Chi Chuan Discourse* refers to the change of void and substantial in shifting weight, striking and so on (see right).

Another Laozi maxim is 'Heavy acts as the root of light; stillness acts as the monarch of the restless.' In *The Canon of Tai Chi Chuan* we have the concept of double-weightedness where there is an absence of Yin

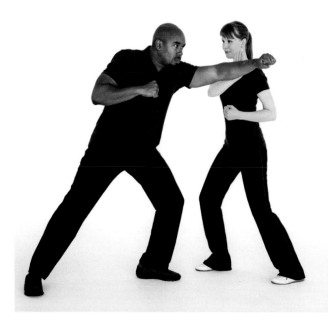

1. She bends her arms in defence.

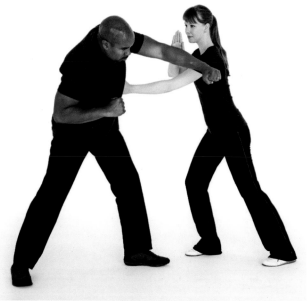

2. Then straightens her arm to counter.

and Yang and therefore an inability to turn and change. What we are aiming at instead is that when heaviness reaches its limit, it reverts to light and vice versa.

Movement and stillness are mentioned a number of times in The Tai Chi Chuan Classics. The point is to move at the right time and to be still at the right time.

As for Laozi's view on the origins of life, 'Something and Nothing give birth to one another', his concept is made flesh in many Tai Chi Hand Forms which begin with a Wu Chi/No Ultimate or At Rest position, then go to a Tai Chi/Supreme Ultimate or Ready Posture.

Laozi mentions 'Return to Wu Chi/the Infinite': this is symbolized at the end of the Tai Chi Form when we move from Tai Chi in Unity to Completion (also known as Wu Chi); so this represents a return to the beginning.

According to Laozi, life is very different from how most people believe it to be. Tai Chi is like this too. 'Tao employs delicacy. The 10,000 things under Heaven are born from Something. Something is born from Nothing.'

Laozi several times mentions the concept of 'Embracing the One/Unity'. 'The Sage embraces the One', for example, refers to the Taoist view that all things

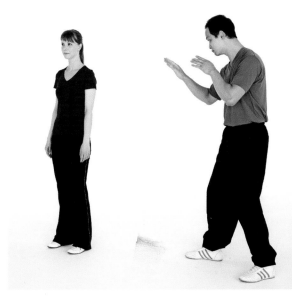

1. Stillness – detecting a threat using peripheral vision.

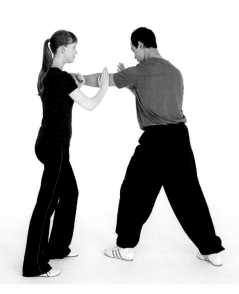

2. Overcoming motion.

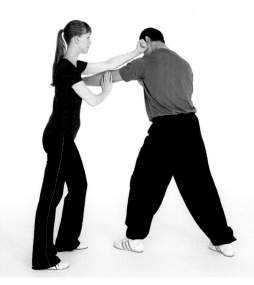

3. Heavy reverts to light, and vice versa.

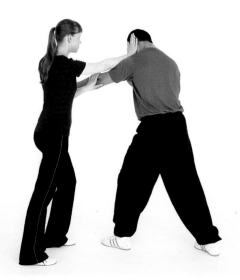

4. Completion.

are fundamentally in unity. It can refer to our life force, the Tao within us. In *The Tai Chi Chuan Discourse*, we chant, 'From the feet to the legs to the waist all must be completely uniform and done in one breath (Qi).'

Laozi hints that if we concentrate our breath, we can be as supple as an infant. In *An Interpretation of the Practice of the 13 Tactics*, we intone, 'From the ability to inhale and exhale properly comes the ability to be nimble and flexible. By constantly developing the Qi there is no evil.'

Laozi advises, 'Deal with a thing while it is still nothing.' *The Fighter's Song* similarly counsels, 'If the opponent doesn't move, I don't move. If the opponent starts to move, I've already moved.'

Laozi goes on, 'Things either move or follow.' In the sequence below, the opponent moved and our Tai Chi lady follows with a pre-emptive strike.

Laozi says,

'The uncarved block is small; under Heaven who dares enable it to be huge?'

and

'If you want something to shrink, you need to lengthen it first. If you want to weaken something, you need to make it stronger first… If you want to take away from something, you first must add to it… The soft and delicate defeats the hard and strong.'

In Tai Chi applications therefore we seek to add to the opponent's force and momentum using body evasion and footwork to unbalance the opponent. If the opponent resists, we add to their resistance by changing our direction of force to go with his resistance (see right).

Likewise, we chant in *The Tai Chi Chuan Discourse*, 'If you raise something up, then there is the intention to smash it down with increased force. In this way its roots will be severed and destruction will be swift and beyond doubt.'

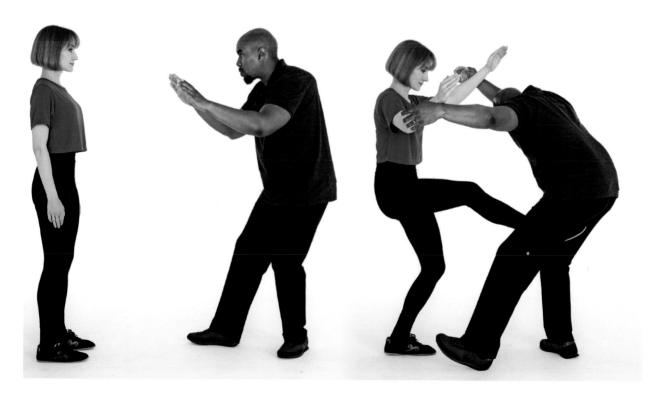

1. She watches him start to move.

2. She follows with a pre-emptive strike.

However, Laozi remains doubtful: 'Delicacy overcomes strength and soft overcomes hard. Under Heaven, there's no-one who doesn't know it, but no-one can do it.'

One of Laozi's recurring themes is Wu Wei, often translated as Inaction or Non-action. For example,

'Tao never acts, but nothing is left undone.'

'The man of the highest virtue doesn't act, yet nothing is left undone.'

'Act without acting.'

This concept is repeated in *The Canon of Tai Chi Chuan* and The Fighter's Song, both of which advise using four taels (Chinese ounces) to displace 1,000 jin (Chinese kilos).

In Tai Chi terms, Wu Wei means avoiding directly opposing the opponent's force, but harmonizing with it instead. This is done by using footwork and body evasion in combination with a defence which leads the opponent's force into emptiness. In the words of *The Canon of Tai Chi Chuan*, 'Other schools of martial arts are so numerous, although there are external differences, yet without exception they amount to nothing more than the strong bullying the weak, the slow surrendering to the fast, the powerful beating those without power, slow hands surrendering to fast hands. This is entirely due to innate ability; it is not related to having learned the skilful use of strength at all.'

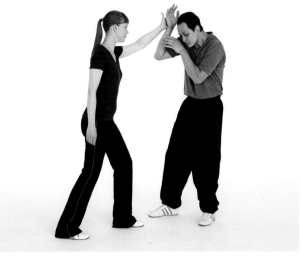

1. He turns to intercept and neutralize his opponent's slap.

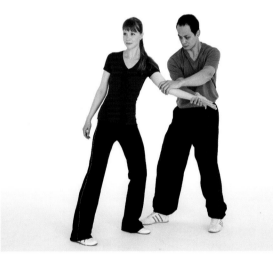

2. He uses her arm to control and unbalance her, changing the direction of force.

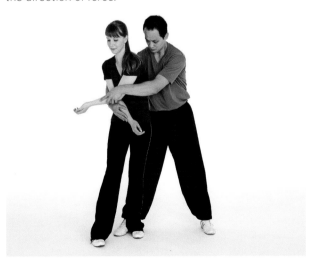

3. He restrains and calms her.

Laozi observes, 'Tao advances, but seems to retreat' and 'Not daring to advance an inch, I retreat a foot instead.' Retreating in order to advance is a famous Chinese military strategy which is often used in Tai Chi self-defence applications (see pages 206–213).
Laozi also has sage advice on fighters and fighting:

'Be careful at the end as at the beginning.'

'If you excel as a warrior, don't seem martial.
If you excel in fighting, don't get angry.'

and

'Being brave and daring leads to death.
Be brave in not daring and you'll live.'

Many years ago, while I was still serving in the Royal Hong Kong Police Force, I was off duty one afternoon waiting for a young lady at the busy Star Ferry Pier in Kowloon. Just then a young Chinese guy came running towards me chased by two other Chinese. He looked back. He tripped and fell. They were on him, stamping and kicking. People just watched. I grabbed one attacker and threw him to the ground and put an arm bar on the other. It was easy.

Suddenly another eight guys came running up, kicking and brawling. I was still using the arm bar and the other

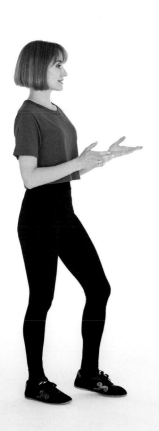

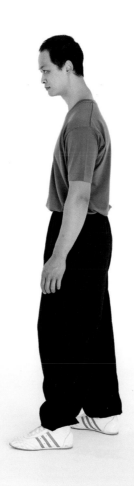

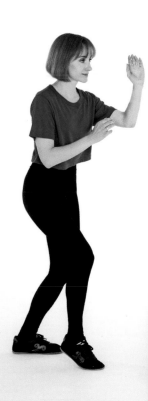

1. She is careful to keep her hands in front of her, to control the distance.

2. She steps back to avoid the attack to her front leg.

two were still down when a smooth-looking Chinese dude came out of the crowd that had gathered and drew an automatic pistol from a shoulder holster. Fortunately, it turned out he was a sergeant from Special Branch. The brawl stopped right then. The sergeant and I got the guys involved to line up in single file with their hands on one another's shoulders and marched them up to nearby Tsimshatsui Police Station, where they got their just deserts. It turned out they were painters working on a boat in the harbour. They started playing cards. You can guess the rest. But I learned something from the experience. I never arrange to meet girls at ferry piers.

Laozi's *The Classic of the Way and Virtue* ends with some beautiful words,

'True words aren't beautiful; beautiful words aren't true.'

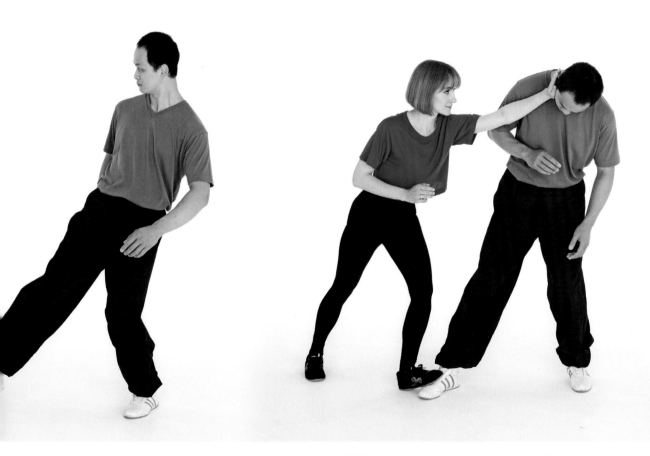

3. She steps back to stamp and palm strike.

Zhuangzi (c. 369–286 BCE)

After Laozi, Zhuangzi is the second most famous Taoist philosopher; his name is also used to refer to his writings. He had similar ideas to Laozi (and therefore Tai Chi theory) on how things began. 'There was a beginning and a beginning before that beginning. There was a beginning before that beginning previous to the beginning.' He goes on, 'It [the Tao] was before the Tai Chi' and

'There was no Nothing and there were no names.'

Zhuangzi talks of balance, knowledge and ability. He ridicules those who 'honour and follow the Yin and take no account of the Yang.' This is a common fault among those who wish to learn Tai Chi for self-defence; their training lacks the Yang element and is not robust enough to be effective.

One of Zhuangzi's best known metaphors is of the Kun fish which lives in the northern darkness and is thousands of li (Chinese kilometres) long. It can change form and become the Peng bird, whose back measures thousands of li across. The Peng rises 90,000 li and flies to the Lake of Heaven in the southern darkness to migrate. The cicadas and doves laugh at the Peng for going so high and so far and wonder why it can't just fly from tree to tree or from branch to branch like them.

The Peng, cicadas and doves are the same in that each is being true to its own nature. However, the Peng represents the Zhenren/True Person and the capacities of cicadas and doves can't be compared to his. It is not for them to judge or understand him. The knowledge of the small is not equal to the knowledge of the great. The knowledge of a few years is not equal to the knowledge of many decades.

'Great knowledge is wide and comprehensive; small knowledge is partial and restricted.'

'There is a limit to our lives, but to knowledge there is no limit.'

We chant in *The Canon of Tai Chi Chuan*, 'It is said a minute discrepancy leads to an error of 1,000 li. The student must carefully discriminate.'

Zhuangzi talks of dexterity acquired by habit, using the analogy of a cook cutting up an ox with a knife. A good cook needs to change his knife every year, an ordinary cook needs to change his knife every month. Zhuangzi's cook has used the same knife for 19 years. It is all a matter of following the Tao when cutting. Acquiring skill in Tai Chi is like this too. In *An Interpretation of the Practice of the 13 Tactics*, we recite, 'Transport the Jin [trained force] like a hundred times refined steel. What firmness can it not break?'

As a reference point Zhuangzi constantly discusses the True Man, the Spiritual Man and the Sage. It seems they are one and the same. He says of the Sage, 'He speaks without speaking.' He acts. In Chinese martial arts, including Tai Chi, there is often little explanation. Sifu does, disciple follows/copies. Some get it, some don't. When fighting, however, we should adopt the zen-like approach of the Sage; it's action, not words that count.

'The breath of a True Man is deep and silent.' This also applies to Tai Chi practice. The True Man is noted for his comprehension of and participation in the Tao.

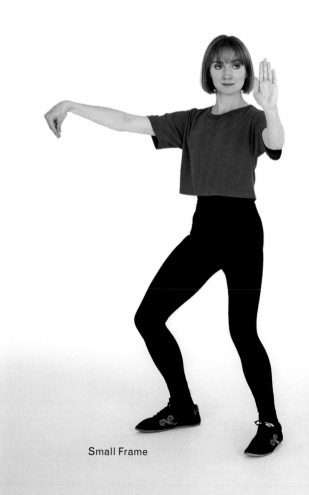

Small Frame

'They [True Men of old] did in regard to all things what was suitable.'

There is a reference in Zhuangzi to man's nine orifices, which may be connected to the passage in *An Interpretation of the Practice of the 13 Tactics* where it is written, 'Move the Qi as through a pearl with nine crooked paths. It goes smoothly everywhere.' Going smoothly is important; Zhuangzi says, 'You must be still; you must be pure and not subject the body to toil; also don't agitate your Qi, then you may have a long life.'

'What's long shouldn't be considered too long, nor what's short too short. It causes pain to try to lengthen a duck's legs and grief to shorten a crane's legs… Now large, now small; now long, now short; now distant, now near.' The point is to do what is appropriate.

Similarly, in *An Interpretation of the Practice of the 13 Tactics*, we recite, 'First seek to expand, then seek to be compact. Thus you will arrive at fine work neatly done.'

Chinese books on Tai Chi Form often refer to Large Frame, Medium Frame and Small Frame.

Large Frame tends to be more expansive and dynamic and looks more martial. It suited big, strong men like Yang Chengfu, the great exponent of Yang lineage Tai Chi, of whom we will hear more later. Small Frame involves tighter, less extended movements and higher stances. It suited those like Wu Yuxiang and his brothers, founders of the Wu lineage, who were a bit older when they took up Tai Chi. Overall my Sifu was Medium Frame, but personally I prefer the feel of Large Frame; when tutoring students for forms competition I emphasize Large Frame as there is more contrast in the movements, making the form more lively.

Some Small Framers make the dubious claim that the smaller the external movement, the greater the internal effect. Easy to say and difficult to prove.

All this relates to form. With regard to application, if movements are too small they'll be ineffective; if they're too large they will be clumsy and slow.

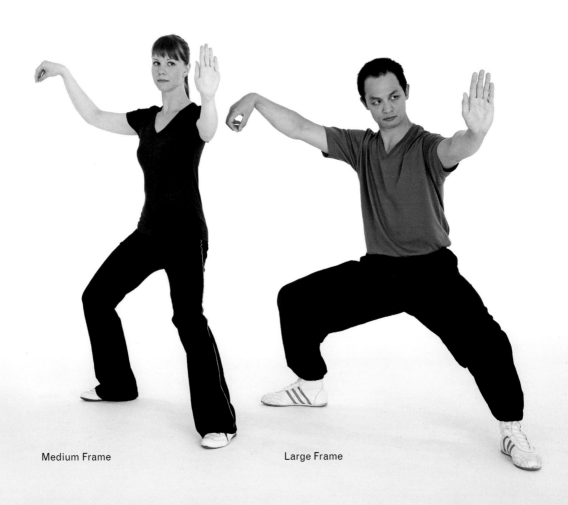

Medium Frame   Large Frame

The Book of Changes

This is the classical Chinese divination text also known as *Yi Jing* or *I Ching*. Appendix II states:

'In the (Book of) Changes is the Tai Chi (Supreme Ultimate/Pole), which produced the Two Principles. The Two Principles produced the Four Emblems, which in turn produced the Eight Trigrams.'

It is often claimed that *Yi Jing* dates back to the beginning of the Zhou dynasty (1122–256 BCE), though modern scholars believe that only the earliest sections may have been written sometime before 1000 BCE. Over the years the text has come to be considered as having a philosophical importance, too. Largely because of its ancient origins, the *Yi Jing* is not seen as a Taoist work, but it greatly influenced both Taoist philosophy and religion, and Tao is discussed in many passages in the book. The key concepts are following the Tao and trying to harmonize the interaction of Yin and Yang and the inevitability of change – essentially the same approach as we should be taking to our Tai Chi practice.

Emperor Fu Xi

The legendary emperor Fu Xi (traditional dates 2800–2737 BCE) is considered to be a kind of Chinese avatar whose vocation was to live among mortal men and be a tutor and advisor for them. He is reputed to have had the Eight Trigrams (Bagua/Pa Kua – see Glossary) revealed to him by a magic tortoise which came out of the river with the trigrams displayed on its shell, each covering one of the Eight Directions. This arrangement of the trigrams is referred to as the River Diagram or the Prior to Heaven Bagua; it is what is referenced in The Tai Chi Chuan Classics and in our Tai Chi practice.

The name of each of the eight forces (below) is is given with its associated trigram. Peng, upward force, is identified with Qian, the trigram for Heaven with three unbroken lines.

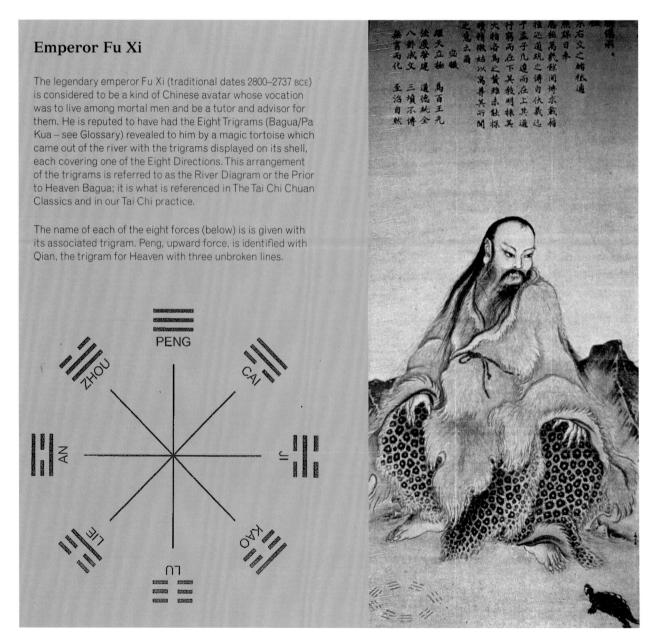

At the end of the Shang dynasty (11th century BCE), King Wen of Zhou is said to have produced an explanation for each hexagram and a descriptive name alluding to its own individual nature. He also came up with a new arrangement of the Eight Trigrams, called the After Heaven Bagua.

Later, after the overthrow of the Shang dynasty, the Duke of Zhou is said to have created explanations for each horizontal line in the hexagrams. It was not until this point that the whole context of the *Yi Jing* was understood. Its philosophy heavily influenced the literature and government administration of the Zhou (1122–256 BCE) and all later dynasties.

The main *Yi Jing* text is now thought to be the work of divinatory soothsayers from the Zhou civilization. The Ten Wings, which sometimes appear as seven appendices and were formerly often attributed to Confucius, are likewise considered to have been written well after his time (the sixth and fifth centuries BCE).

The main text is a series of oracular pronouncements relating to each of the 64 hexagrams. Each hexagram is composed of six stacked horizontal lines; each line is either Yin or Yang, with Yin symbolized by a broken line and Yang by an unbroken one. These lines represent the vagina and the penis and thus female and male,

soft and hard, internal and external, and a host of other complementary opposites. These two single lines are called the Two Principles.

From the single broken and unbroken lines we can produce two pairs of double lines, known as the Four Emblems. The Four Emblems comprise Old Yin, Young Yang, Young Yin and Old Yang. In turn the Four Emblems produce the Eight Trigrams, which can be matched up to produce the 64 hexagrams. The trigrams and hexagrams were used as metaphors for directions, animals, natural phenomena and so on. In Tai Chi, each of the Eight Forces is seen as being linked to a specific trigram.

There are various methods of consulting the *Yi Jing*; all involve selection of the appropriate hexagram(s) and identifying the relevant lines in the text. Traditionally, consulting the *Yi Jing* was taken seriously; prior to consulting it, supplicants would go through three days of fast and abstinence, bathe from head to toe and wear clean clothing before daring to start their consultation. No-one does this any more.

Some Tai Chi teachers have tried to correlate specific Tai Chi techniques with specific hexagrams, for example, as in the book entitled *T'ai Chi Ch'uan and I Ching* by the late Da Liu. It wasn't convincing when it was published, more than 40 years ago, and it isn't convincing now.

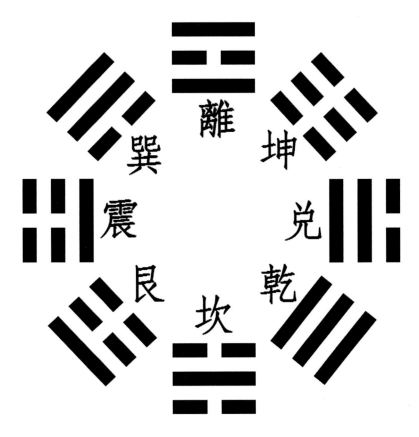

Right After heaven Bagua.

Calligraphy

In the *Yi Jing* there are three main terms meaning 'change', the first being the character **Yi** in the title. This depicts a lizard, probably the chameleon, and by extension derives its core meanings of to change and to transform; it can also mean easy.

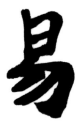

The second word for change, which appears repeatedly in the text of the *Yi Jing*, is **Bian**. The upper part of the character for Bian depicts a hand untangling threads. Change can take a bit of effort. Bian is also used in *The Song of the 13 Tactics*, to refer to the necessity of maintaining the intent during the changes of void and substantial.

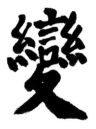

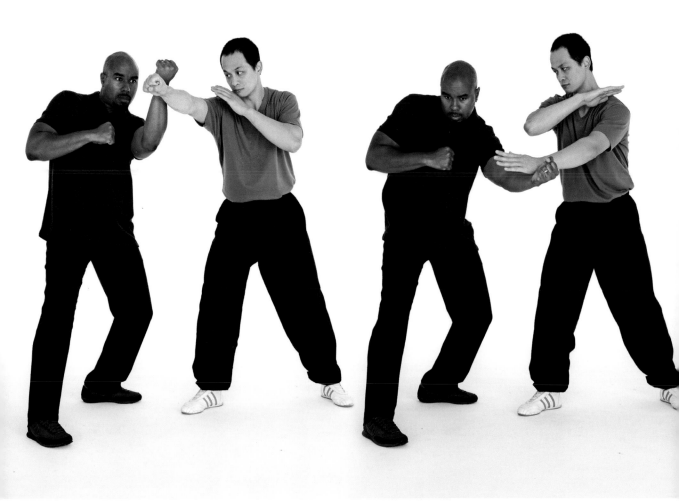

1. Yi: The opponent's punch is blocked.

2. Bian: The right opponent relaxes, bringing his arms around in an arc, following the left opponent's force.

The third symbol for change, **Hua**, often translated as 'to transform or convert', is a drawing of person(s) and men. It appears in *The Canon of Tai Chi Chuan*, where the inability to 'turn and change' indicates the sickness of double-weightedness.

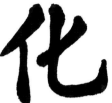

Sometimes, for emphasis, the compound term Bian Hua is used: in *The Song of the 13 Tactics*, it refers to the practitioner's changes being in accordance with those of the opponent and appearing mysterious. It also appears in *The Canon of Tai Chi Chuan*: 'Though there are 10,000 transformations, the principle remains the same.'

The *Yi Jing*, when it advises action, normally suggests that such action be harmonious. In Taoism this was to become the doctrine of Oneness, much discussed by Laozi.

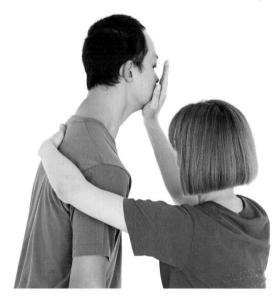

1. She tries to bend him back with Pat the Horse High (see page 139), but he resists.

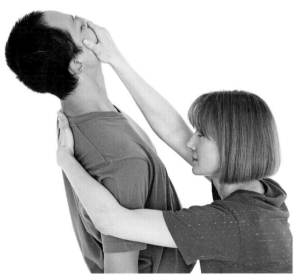

2. She moves her right hand so she is directly attacking the philtrum (vital point below the nostrils).

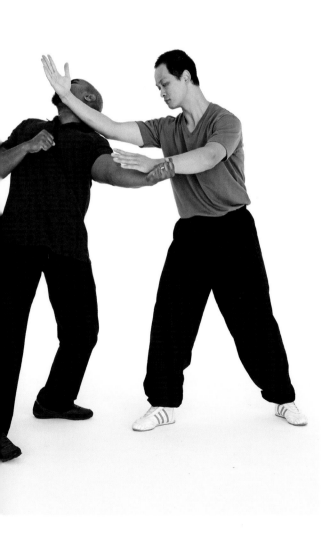

3. Hua: The right opponent counters to his opponent's head.

Recurring dualities in the *Yi Jing* include hard and soft, above and below, (see below) and advancing and retreating as appropriate. These are all also recurring themes in The Tai Chi Chuan Classics and are to be found in Tai Chi forms, in Pushing Hands and above all in martial applications.

A key character in the text is Zhong, meaning centre or central. It depicts a target pierced by an arrow through the centre. Even today the Chinese refer to their country as Zhongguo, the Central Kingdom, reflecting their world and cultural view.

Another key character is Zheng, which means correct or straight, both in a physical and in a moral sense. The character depicts the feet stopping when they reach the level/limit at the top. From a Tai Chi perspective at least, it's great when you're straight.

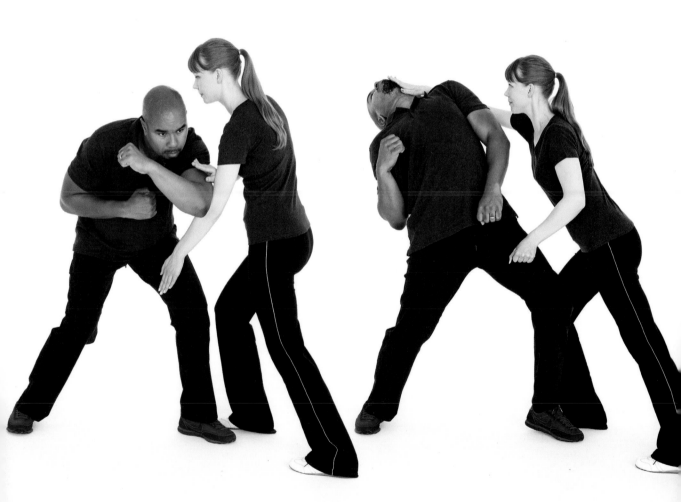

Recurring dualities in the Yi Jing: Hard and soft.　　　　Above and below.

The compound term Zhongzheng, meaning centrally correct, normally in a moral/psychological context, also appears frequently in the *Yi Jing*. The Tai Chi Classics apply this term both to the body structure and to the psychological mindset of the practitioner (see below).

The Interpretation of the Practice of the 13 Tactics says, 'When standing, the body should be Zhongzheng and at ease to deal with attacks from the Eight Directions.' Incorrect alignment adversely affects the balance, coordination and speed of reaction.

The Song of the 13 Tactics states, 'When the coccyx is Zhongzheng, the Shen [Spirit] ascends to the headtop. The whole body feels light and agile when the headtop is suspended.' Incorrect alignment adversely affects the functioning of the central nervous system, which runs through the spinal column.

In the *Yi Jing* it is written, 'I don't seek the youthful and inexperienced, they come and seek me.' This is how it was when my Sifu met his Sifu. My Sifu was a 16-year-old country boy from a village in Guangdong province; his Sifu was an austere man from Henan province and spoke a different dialect. For almost three years they roamed all over Hong Kong together, then the older man left for home. They never met again. It's how it was when I met my Sifu, too. He was a fat, irascible, chain-smoker with a sense of humour. He couldn't speak English.

We got along just fine. Neither of us had wanted to learn from just anybody; we chose our masters carefully. Unfortunately many Sifu and their students don't take care over this and become bound in chains of ignorance.

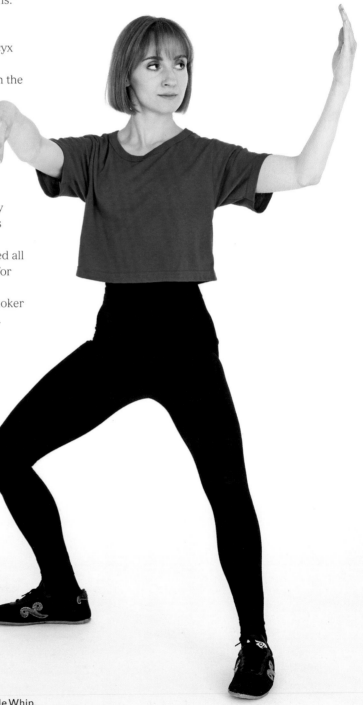

Centrally correct: She stays erect as she turns into Single Whip.

The hexagram Yu represents satisfaction and harmony; the next hexagram in sequence is Sui, meaning to follow. *The Fighter's Song* refers to being in harmony with the opponent's attack. The strategy of following is also referred to in The Tai Chi Chuan Classics: following in the sense of deferring or seeming to defer to others both verbally and through body language is one of the big games of Chinese culture and one of the great games of Tai Chi too (see below).

Hexagram 26 of the *Yi Jing*, Great Accumulation, recommends daily practice of charioteering and methods of defence. Mobility training, including footwork and evasion, is vital in Tai Chi too; many practitioners neglect it.

Yin and Yang are of equal importance in their various interactions; according to Appendix I of the *Yi Jing*, 'Heaven and earth are separate and apart, but the work that they do is the same.'

According to Appendix II, 'A one-eyed man can see, but isn't fit to see clearly.' This admonition is relevant for Tai Chi tutors and Tai Chi trainees alike. Every aspect of Tai Chi is interrelated, so if you want to understand it properly, you need to learn and to practise a complete system.

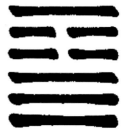

Above Hexagram 26 of the *Yi Jing*.

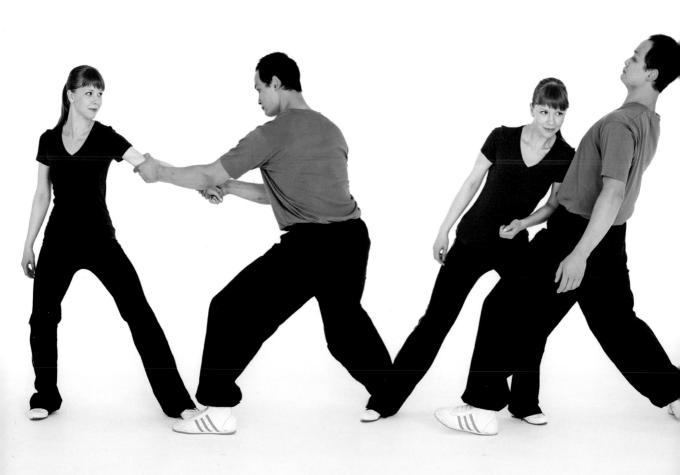

Pretending to resist

Following the opponent's force.

Hua Tuo (c. 140–208 CE)

Besides being a famous physician, respected for expertise in surgery and anaesthesia, Hua Tuo was known for his abilities in acupuncture, moxibustion, herbal medicine and medical Daoyin/Leading and Conducting exercises. He developed the Five Animal Frolic or Exercise of the Five Animals from studying movements of the tiger, deer, bear, ape and bird.

Hua Tuo is said to have told his student Wu Pu that our bodies need exercise, but that it shouldn't be excessive. Moving the limbs helps us to absorb nutrients in food and enhances blood circulation, thus preventing all kinds of illness. The exercises involve constant opening and closing. When practising, the adept walks like a bear and twists his head back like an owl. He stretches the waist and limbs and manipulates all of their joints, seeking to prevent the infirmities of old age. Practising the exercises can eradicate sickness and is good for circulation in the legs and feet. If your body doesn't feel at ease, get up and practise at least one of the Five Animal exercises until you're perspiring. The body will become more relaxed and your appetite will improve.

Chen Tuan (906–89 CE)

This mysterious Taoist scholar hermit lived a secluded life in the Nine Room Cave on Wudang Mountain, before going to Huashan, where he is said to have invented the internal martial art of Six Harmonies and Eight Methods. On the cliffs at Huashan, Chen is supposed to have carved out his Wu Chi/No Ultimate Diagram. Here, too, he's said to have defeated the Emperor at a game of chess, winning the mountain for Taoism. A pavilion now marks the spot where the game traditionally took place. Chen is also credited with creating the Tai Chi Ruler Qigong training and a 24-exercise Daoyin/Leading and Conducting Qigong to help exponents adjust to seasonal changes throughout the year. Known as the 'Sleeping Immortal', he is supposed to have practised sleeping Qigong involving internal alchemy. He heavily influenced the Tai Chi Diagram Sect.

Zhou Dunyi (1017–73 CE)

Zhou was the most outstanding representative of the Neo-Confucian school of philosophy which re-interpreted the major ancient philosophical texts in an attempt to answer the burning question of the age concerning man and his place in the cosmic order. Specifically, he was a member of the Tai Chi Diagram Sect, one of three Taoist sects which trace their origin from the great Chen Tuan. We can see from the diagram that Zhou was concerned with Five Element theory as well as with Yin/Yang theory. Unsurprisingly, he was an adept of Taoist internal alchemy. I would be astonished if he were the only Neo-Confucian / Tai Chi Diagram Sect adherent with such a proclivity.

The Tai Chi Diagram of Zhou Dunyi (see page 32) is effectively a simplified version of the Chinese system of cosmogony (for their theory about the origins of the universe – see page 15). Starting from the top we have Wu Chi yet Tai Chi. Tao and Tai Chi must come from that which is not – Wu Chi – but if there is Wu Chi then there must also paradoxically be Tai Chi. We can see the concept of Wu Chi (No Pole/Ultimate) as being a Taoist one and the concept of Tai Chi (Supreme Pole/Ultimate) as being Confucian. The Confucians sought order in the universe, in society and in the individual, so the idea of a fixed point such as the Pole Star as a sort of centre from which order in the universe stemmed was very attractive. The Taoists were more concerned with harmonious change, so the idea that there was no one fixed pole, Wu Chi, but instead constant change, made perfect sense. The statement 'Wu Chi yet Tai Chi' reconciles these different approaches.

Below the empty Tai Chi circle we have the concentric half-Yin, half-Yang circles, in which the Yang manifests itself in motion. When this reaches its limit, it is followed by Yin, which is manifest in stillness; when stillness has reached its limit, there is a return to movement. In this way, movement and stillness, Yin and Yang, each in turn becomes the source of the other. This is precisely what happens in Tai Chi form, in Pushing Hands and in self-defence.

The interaction of Yin and Yang produces the Five Elements of Metal, Wood, Water, Fire and Earth.

Water is largely Yin and is on the right, while Fire is largely Yang and is on the left. Wood produces Fire and is also on the left, while Metal produces Water (in the form of condensation) and is also on the right. Earth is of mixed nature, so is fixed in the centre. The crossed lines above Fire and Water show Yin generating Yang and vice versa.

The Five Elements can operate in either a generative or a destructive cycle. In the generative cycle, Metal produces Water; Water produces Wood; Wood produces Fire; Fire produces Earth; Earth produces Metal. This is in accord with Nature and can also be represented by the clockwise-rotating Tai Chi symbol. In the destructive cycle Metal destroys Wood; Wood destroys Earth; Earth destroys Water; Water destroys Fire; Fire destroys Metal. This is contrary to Nature and can be represented by the anti-clockwise-rotating Tai Chi symbol.

According to Yin/Yang theory, each element is stronger than two of the other elements and weaker than the other two. Furthermore, each element individually has Yin and Yang

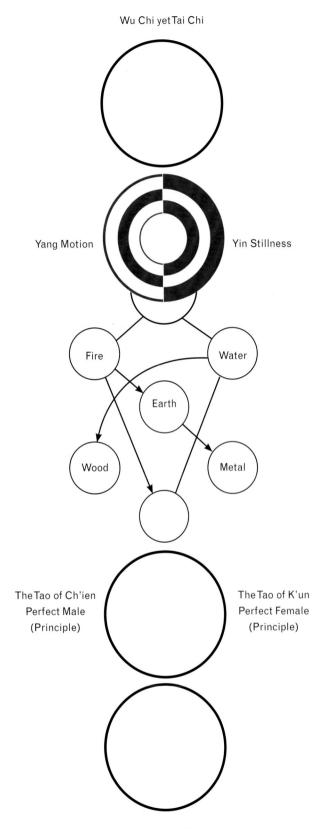

Wu Chi yet Tai Chi

Yang Motion   Yin Stillness

Fire   Water

Earth

Wood   Metal

The Tao of Ch'ien
Perfect Male
(Principle)

The Tao of K'un
Perfect Female
(Principle)

The Ten Thousand Things are
transformed and produced

aspects. Thus Metal could be shiny or rusty. Water could be a puddle or a vast river.

The small circle below the Five Elements and joined to them by four lines again represents Wu Chi where they unite (see left).

The first large circle below the Five Elements represents on the left the Tao of Heaven, which perfects maleness; on the right it represents the Tao of Earth, which perfects femaleness. The two Qi of maleness and femaleness interact and complement one another, bringing them back to the one Tai Chi (Supreme Pole).

The final circle represents the birth of the Ten Thousand Things, caused by the interaction of the male and female principles and their return to the one Tai Chi. Some 3,000 years after these concepts and terms first appeared we are still applying them in Tai Chi Chuan.

Zhu Xi (1130–1200 CE)

A scholar/official who was influenced by the Tai Chi Diagram Sect and followed the Neo-Confucian tradition, Zhu was given imperial honours after his death. Today, he is venerated as one of the 12 Philosophers of Confucianism.

During his lifetime, Zhu Xi's teachings were considered unorthodox. Rather than focusing on *Yi Jing* like other Neo-Confucians, he emphasized the Four Books: *The Great Learning, The Doctrine of the Mean, The Analects of Confucius* and *Mencius*; his detailed commentaries on these works became the standard after his death.

Zhu Xi believed that the union of Qi and Li (principles/law) brings all things into being. Li comes from the Tai Chi, the Supreme Ultimate, the energy behind the operation of the universe. All physical objects, including people, have Li and are thereby connected to Tai Chi. The human soul, mind or spirit is understood as everyone's personal Tai Chi. Zhu Xi claimed these concepts came from *The Book of Changes*.

He also believed that the task of moral cultivation is to clear our Qi. If our Qi is clear and balanced, then we will act in a moral way. Perhaps this is why Zhu Xi engaged in Jingzuo/quiet sitting meditation.

Left The Tai Chi Diagram of Zhou Dunyi.

The Seven Military Classics

This collection of essays on military strategy was written between 500 BCE and 700 CE; the most famous is the '13 Chapters on Employing Troops' by Sunzi (c. 544–496 BCE). Many of the topics covered in these essays – such as situations to avoid, probing and manipulating the enemy, terrain, escape from entrapment, attacking when and where the enemy is unprepared, changing and transforming from orthodox to unorthodox and back again, and deception – are also relevant in Tai Chi self-defence. The ultimate aim is the same: to maximize results with minimum risk and exposure to oneself. The strategist Sunzi considered subjugating the enemy without fighting to be the highest skill.

In his writings Sunzi tells the story of the Shuaijan, a snake found on the peak of Mount Chang. If you attacked the tail, the head responded; if you attacked the body, both head and tail responded. The idea is to use both top and bottom and to have one technique following another in combination. The techniques can be for real or just feints – in Tai Chi parlance, full or empty. This story was later quoted by General Qi Jiguang (1528–87 CE) in his *Classic of Boxing*, although largely unconnected with the theory expounded in The Tai Chi Chuan Classics (see page 51 where the links between Tai Chi and *The Classic of Boxing* are discussed). Elsewhere Sunzi advises feinting and attacking where the opponent is unprepared or empty. In Tai Chi self-defence we also use feints and hit where the opponent is open.

The Tai Chi Chuan Discourse says, 'Void and substantial must be clearly distinguished. Each place has its individual balance of void and substantial. Every place consists of this, one void and substantial.' Sunzi advises, 'Avoid the substantial and strike the void.'

He also states, 'If you know yourself and know the enemy, a hundred battles will result in a hundred victories. If you know yourself, but don't know the enemy, you'll sometimes be victorious and sometimes be defeated. If you know neither yourself nor the enemy, you'll always be defeated.'

The Song of the 13 Tactics paraphrases Sunzi thus, 'In accordance with the opponent, my changes appear mysterious.'

Tai Chi Chuan is essentially a counter-attacking martial art. We detect what the opponent is doing and respond immediately.

Below A name tablet of Sunzi former residence.

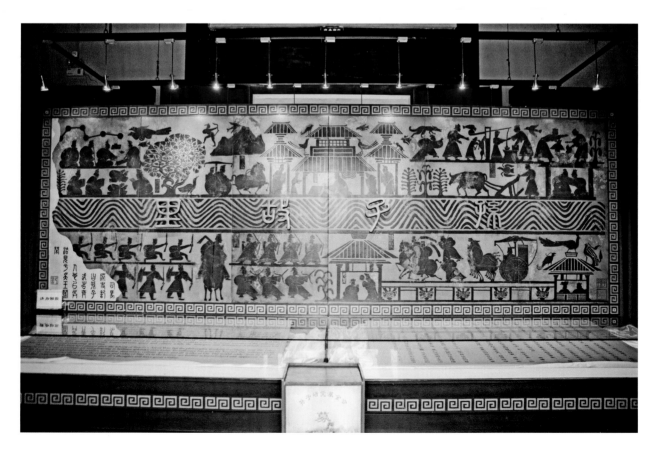

Tai Gong's Six Secret Teachings

The strategist Tai Gong is said to have lived in the 11th century BCE, but the text known as Tai Gong's Six Secret Teachings probably dates from the time of the Warring States (475–221 BCE). It mentions that a king's army needs 'arms and legs' (top officials) and 'feathers and wings' (aides). The body, too, is like an army. According to *The Tai Chi Chuan Discourse*, 'In particular it [the body] must be linked together.'

Tai Gong's list of errors that generals should avoid includes 'being courageous and treating death lightly, being hasty and impatient, being benevolent but unwilling to inflict suffering, being wise but fearful, being trustworthy and liking to trust others, being wise but indecisive'. The same errors apply when using Tai Chi for self-defence, but can be overcome by training.

The samurai in Old Japan practised Zen, painted and studied calligraphy as well as training in the martial arts, because they believed these activities would help them to develop the key skill of harmonious spontaneity. Practice of the more Yin aspects of Tai Chi and the unpredictable nature of free Pushing Hands training similarly help to develop that spontaneity. Tai Gong goes on to say:

'He who excels in warfare will await events in the situation without making any movement. If he sees he can be victorious, he'll arise.'

'He who excels in warfare won't lose an advantage when he perceives it, or be doubtful when he meets the moment.'

Both these quotes relate to timeliness. Similar advice can be found in *The Fighter's Song*.

The Three Strategies of Huang Shigong, also attributed to Tai Gong, is a text dating from around the 1st century. It says, 'One who abandons what is nearby to plan for what is distant will labour without success.' In *The Canon of Tai Chi Chuan* it is written, 'Many err by forsaking what is near to pursue what is far.' The essential message is to deal with what immediately needs to be done; to choose the nearest target.

The text continues, 'The soft can control the hard; the weak can control the strong.' *The Canon of Tai Chi Chuan* has it, 'When the opponent is hard and stiff and I am pliant and soft, this is called Zou [moving].' When you are hard and stiff you use up more energy than if you were soft and it's difficult to change what you're doing; you end up being controlled by others.

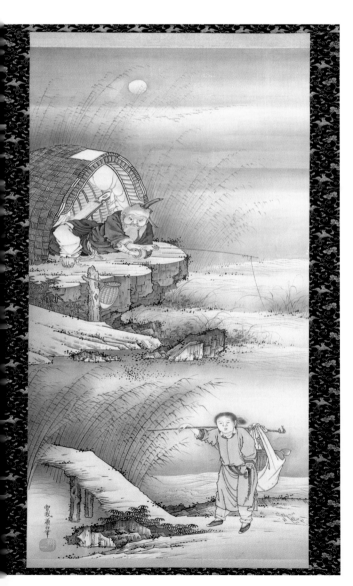

Left When King Wen of Zhou (11th century BCE) went to recruit Tai Gong, he found him fishing without a hook – the fish gave up when they were ready. Tai Gong Fishing is also the name of a Tai Chi sword technique.

The Yellow Emperor's Canon of Internal Medicine

Believed to have been compiled between the late Warring States period (475–221 BCE) and the early Han dynasty (206 BCE–220 CE), this seminal Chinese medical text includes advice such as:

• 'If we are free from desires, the true Qi will come. When we concentrate the vitality [Jingshen] internally and stay at ease, how can there be sickness?' Focusing on your Tai Chi practice will relax you and help you to forget your worries.

• 'Zhenren [True Persons] inhale and exhale the Jing and Qi and guard the spirit…so they can live long.' Those who have become at one with the Tao by training and developing their breath and circulation, body essences and spirit will thereby lengthen their lifespans.

• The Yellow Emperor, like Zhuangzi, states, 'Man has nine orifices'. He advises that the orifices must be kept clear of internal obstruction or there will be an adverse effect on the Qi. In addition to correct practice, environment and basic hygiene are important.

Violent mood swings damage the internal organs and the Qi. Regular Tai Chi practice has a soothing effect on mind and body, helping us to control our emotions instead of being controlled by them.

• 'When you know how to regulate Yin and Yang properly, the body will be strong. When you don't know how to regulate Yin and Yang, the body will become decrepit and senile.'

In *The Song of the 13 Tactics* we chant, 'Think and enquire where does the final purpose lie? It lies in seeking longevity and keeping a youthful appearance.' In Tai Chi practice, as in life, harmony and change are vital.

• 'The mind is the supreme commander/monarch of the body.' The Chinese believe that it is the heart that does all the thinking.

This observation resonates in two of The Tai Chi Chuan Classics. In *An Interpretation of the Practice of the 13 Tactics* we have, 'The mind is the commander', while in *The Song of the 13 Tactics* we find, 'Yi and Qi are the rulers' and other vital organs are compared to different officials.

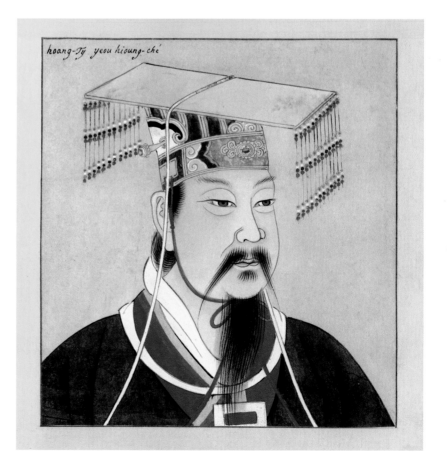

Right The Yellow Emperor.

Into the Unknown

This section analyses the connections between relatively well-known mainstream ancient Chinese literary works and Tai Chi. Many of the links are little known even among Chinese people. It also presents other relevant sources such as the concept of Nei Ye/Inward Training, the writings of Heguanzi and *The Book of Balance and Harmony*, which are more obscure and clearly part of the 'lost' Tai Chi.

The Known Unknowns

Confucianism was what the Chinese used to call one of the Three Teachings – the others being Buddhism and Taoism. Although the Taoist contribution to Tai Chi is perhaps better known, the Confucian tradition is just as important although perhaps less well understood. Principles linked to Tai Chi can found in the ideas of key Confucian thinkers.

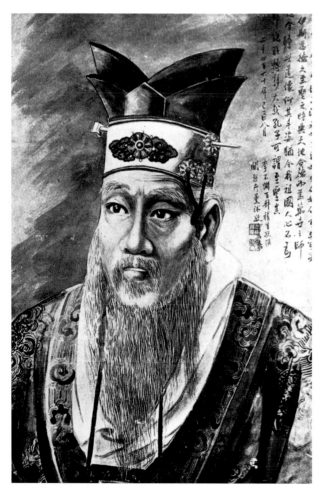

The Book of Odes

The oldest existing collection of Chinese poetry, *The Book of Odes* dates from the 11th to the 7th centuries BCE and is one of the Five Classics traditionally said to have been compiled by Confucius (551–479 BCE). In the poems there are brief references to silent meditation, to the Tao and to duality. All these themes are now aspects of Tai Chi.

'The black-eared kite flies and the fish leaps' expresses how discoveries are made from both above and below. It is also the name of one of the techniques of the Spear Form which I teach, though in this case the metaphor is martial.

The Analects of Confucius

Confucius said, 'At 15, my mind was bent on learning.' Li Bai (701–62), the famous poet and knight errant, once mischievously wrote, 'At 15 I loved the sword.'

Confucius is seen as a great sage and a great teacher. He travelled around with a group of disciples trying to educate them in correct behaviour and to pass on his doctrines. Confucius left no writings behind; the Analects were compiled by his disciples. Like Confucius, as a teenager, my Sifu roamed all over the hills and islands of Hong Kong, learning Tai Chi from his Sifu.

Confucius said that he didn't want anyone with him who'd attack a tiger unarmed or try to cross a river without a boat, dying without regret. People like this are not suitable for learning Tai Chi either. *The Canon of Tai Chi Chuan* tells us, 'You can often see folk who've been practising their skills for several years, but who still can't change and turn. This leads to their being entirely regulated by others. They aren't aware of their sickness of double-weightedness. To be free from this sickness, they must know Yin and Yang.'

'I conceal nothing from you,' Confucius once said.

Left The great teacher Confucius.
Right Confucius sharing his wisdom with his disciples.

In Chinese martial arts, including Tai Chi, the opposite is often true. My teacher's uncle was even worse: rather than refuse to teach people, he'd teach them wrongly. I remember the look of horror on the face of one of my Tai Chi uncles from Malaysia when I explained that he'd been practising Running Thunder Hand incorrectly for more than 20 years.

Confucius had a serious attitude to learning: 'Some don't know, yet they act. I'm not like that. Hear more; select and follow the useful. See more; and remember it.'

This is paraphrased in *The Canon of Tai Chi Chuan*:

'Silently memorize, study and imitate. Gradually we reach the point where we can do all we wish.'

Yen Yuan, a disciple of Confucius, said of his master's doctrines, 'Looking up, they're higher still. In trying to penetrate them, they become firmer. Looking forward at them, suddenly they're behind me.'

Similarly, *The Canon of Tai Chi Chuan* tells us:

'Suddenly conceal, suddenly reveal.'

'When the opponent looks up, I am still higher. When he looks down, I'm lower still.'

Confucius advised,

'When you have faults, don't be afraid to reform.'

Even when Tai Chi faults have been corrected, it is difficult for the student to change as there is a muscle memory of practising the fault. The best remedy is to practise more slowly so you can consciously absorb the correction.

The *Analects of Confucius* describe Confucius using the appropriate body language in different situations and in different company. This is a key skill and in my experience women are better at it than men. Good body language

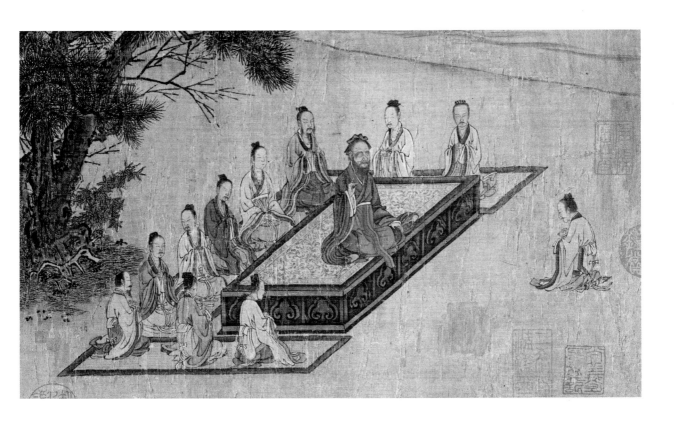

can make a difficult situation better. Inappropriate body language can make things much worse. I used to teach Management of Aggression courses to security guards and hospital staff. Body language was part of the syllabus. Tai Chi practice will improve the posture. Better posture leads to better body language.

Confucius said a man may be able to recite *The Book of Odes*, but if he doesn't know how to discharge his duties and is unable to take questions, of what practical use is his learning? Likewise, a lot of Tai Chi people do nice-looking forms, and can quote The Tai Chi Chuan Classics, but don't know how to apply them.

'To use an uninstructed people in war is throwing them away.' And yet I've seen well-known Tai Chi instructors put their students into Chinese full-contact fighting with little or no preparation and watch those students take awful beatings.

Confucius advocated reciprocity; he said, 'Treat injury with justice and treat kindness with kindness.' Good advice for a Tai Chi tutor.

The Great Learning

The Confucian classic *The Great Learning* was the work of many authors and was written in the 5th century BCE.

Learning Tai Chi is a mission. *The Great Learning* tells us, 'We need to know where we want to end up, We need to be clear what our mission is, then we can be still and in calmness execute that mission.'

The text has sound observations on the correct approach: 'Once we examine things our knowledge becomes complete.'

Likewise in *The Song of the 13 Tactics* we chant, 'Be meticulous and keep the mind on enquiring into the art.'

'With our root in chaos, its branches can't be in order.' *The Tai Chi Chuan Discourse* tells us, 'The root is in the feet.' The aim of being rooted is to be better balanced in applying techniques. So in all types of training we strive to keep the centre of gravity low to develop this skill.

Elsewhere in this book we discuss the benefits of regular practice; *The Great Learning* suggests, 'If you can renew yourself one day, do it every day.'

The Song of the 13 Tactics similarly advises, 'Kung Fu is unceasing. Cultivate the method yourself.'

Zhong Yong/The Doctrine of the Mean

The two-character term Zhong Yong is both a philosophical concept in its own right and the title of one of the Confucian Classics (Zhong meaning centre or centrality, Yong meaning stability or control). The Classic is what we are discussing here. It was written around 400 BCE and is attributed to Confucius' grandson Zisi. Although the English title is most commonly given as

The Doctrine of the Mean, a more accurate translation is *The Doctrine of Centrality* [*Zhong*] and *Constancy* [*Yong*]. It means that one is focused and emotionally detached and behaves appropriately in a particular set of circumstances according to one's nature and code. This may require minimal effort or action or an extreme amount of effort or action. In fact many of the admonitions of *The Doctrine of the Mean* are as difficult to follow as those of the Good Book.

One of the most telling quotations from *The Doctrine of the Mean* is:

'If others do it once and can achieve it, I will do it a hundred times If others do it ten times and can achieve it, I will do it a thousand times'

In order to achieve Zhong Yong, constant and repeated effort is required. Zhong Yong is also the answer to more than 90 per cent of the questions asked in Tai Chi classes. When students ask me how big their movements should be, I tell them, 'Not too big, not too small'. When they ask how fast they should practise the sword, I tell them, 'Not too fast, not too slow.' When they ask how many back bends to do, I tell them, 'Not more than 360.' When they ask how much punching with weights they should do, I tell them, 'Not more than 20 minutes.' These answers could all be described as Zhong Yong.

Externally someone's level of Zhong Yong is evidenced by their behaviour, internally by their integrity. As martial artists we can judge the former in the technique and spirit of an individual, both of which are forged by repetitive training.

I remember an interesting conversation I had many years ago with the owner of a taverna in Crete. Amazed at my gargantuan appetite, he told me this story. Once upon a time a stranger went into a taverna and ordered 99 souvlaki. The astounded taverna owner said, 'Ninety-nine souvlaki! Why not go all the way and order a hundred?' The stranger replied, 'Who can eat a hundred souvlaki?'

The point is that there are both limits and targets; with time and effort we can expand those limits and hit those targets. One of my heroes is Mr Wong Seung-yau, a small, tubby Tai Chi practitioner in Hong Kong. Mr Wong is in his eighties; he's not a fighter, his Tai Chi isn't even particularly good, but he is still my hero.

This is because in 1988, when I was preparing to give a Tai Chi seminar in Australia with my Sifu, I noticed that

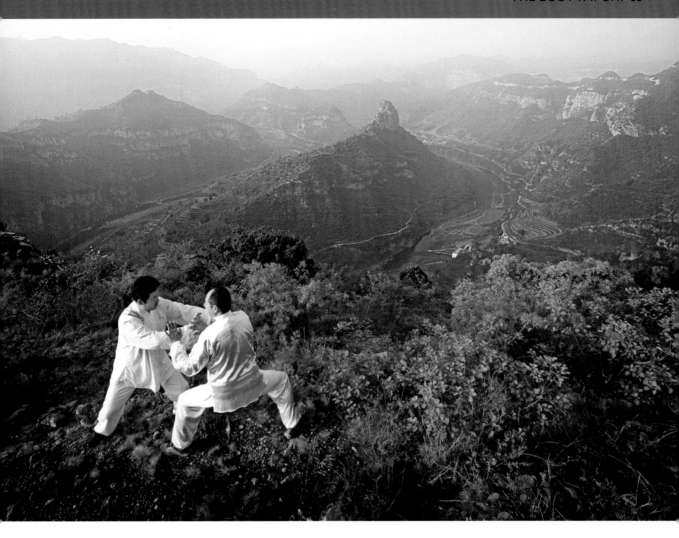

every lunchtime Mr Wong would come up to the rooftop training area and practise the Sabre Form over and over again. I remarked that I didn't understand why he needed to practise the Sabre so much when he'd been doing Tai Chi for more than 30 years.

He said that, like me, he would be demonstrating at a forthcoming Tai Chi banquet. He dared not lose face in front of the younger people there by not having the energy necessary to demonstrate the Sabre at the correct speed, so for the last two weeks he had been practising the Sabre Form 20 times in an hour every day.

Mr Wong knows Zhong Yong. Mr Wong is a true martial hero. Mr Wong did a good demo on the night. But I don't know if Mr Wong could eat 99 souvlaki, never mind a hundred.

The Doctrine of the Mean continues: 'Not leaning to one side or the other is called Centrality. Not changing is called Constancy. Centrality is the correct way (Tao) for all under Heaven. Constancy is the fixed rule for all under Heaven.'

Above Pushing hands practise in the misty mountains.

The Canon of Tai Chi Chuan likewise (but from a physical rather than metaphorical viewpoint) advises, 'Empty the neck and headtop of strength. The Qi sinks to the Dantian/Cinnabar Field. Don't lean to either side or forward or back.' The Cinnabar Field is a concept from internal alchemy. It divides the Dantian into three fields, with the Cinnabar, which is connected with sexual energy and regeneration, just below the navel. The point here is that the headtop, neck, spine and Dantian must be aligned during form practice if the body is to work efficiently.

Being centred and acting in harmony with your surroundings are two of the great themes of *The Doctrine of the Mean*: 'Centrality is the great root of all under Heaven; Harmony is the suitable way (Tao) of all under Heaven.'

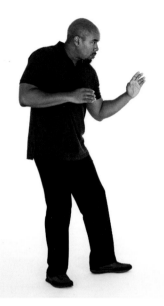
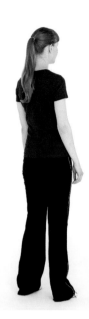
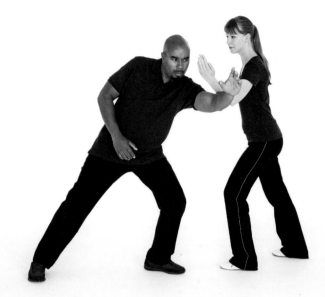

1. Her peripheral vision detects a threat.

2. She swings round to avoid and intercept.

Similarly from *The Fighter's Song* we chant, 'Lead the opponent into the void, harmonize and immediately discharge.' In other words, avoid and control the opponent's attack and immediately counter him (see above).

A violent thug who was later dismissed from the Royal Hong Kong Police Force once made the mistake of trying to kick me in the groin in the officers' mess. I sidestepped and scooped up his kicking leg, harmonizing with and adding to his force; he became briefly airborne and landed on his coccyx. He was not okay. I had to get some others to help me lift him into an armchair.

The Doctrine of the Mean leaves us in no doubt about what is expected:

'The superior man is centred and constant, the small man is not.'

'When an archer misses the bulls-eye, he turns and looks for the cause of his failure in himself.'

So, chanting *The Canon of Tai Chi Chuan*, 'The more we train, the more expert we become.'

Mencius (372–289 BCE)

The philosopher Mencius is second only to Confucius himself in importance in the Confucian school. *Mencius* is also the name we give to his collected 'conversations'.

'Those who toil with their minds control others; those who toil with their strength are controlled by others.'

This is precisely what we are trying to do with Tai Chi – evade, redirect, unbalance and counter the opponent. Mencius made valid points on teaching:

'The evil of men is that they like to act as the teacher of others'

and

'If I refuse to teach a man, am I not thereby still teaching him?'

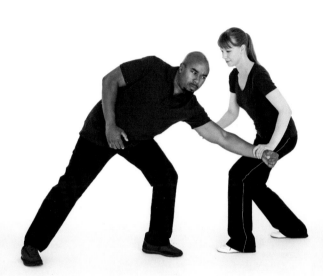

3. She tries to lead the opponent into emptiness.

4. When he resists she changes to a punch.

A great many Tai Chi teachers are not really very good; they need a tutor. I have to agree with Mencius. If people offend me, I don't refuse to teach them; I prefer to ignore them. It's another kind of teaching.

Mencius said that shooting an arrow and reaching a mark a thousand paces away is due to strength; actually hitting the mark is not. Mencius wasn't wrong. We need strength to deliver Tai Chi techniques and skill to target them.

Mencius' view on philosophy trolls is an accurate picture of Tai Chi Internet trolls too: 'Man's sickness is that he neglects his own fields, but goes to weed the fields of others. What they seek from others is heavy; the pressure they put on themselves is light.'

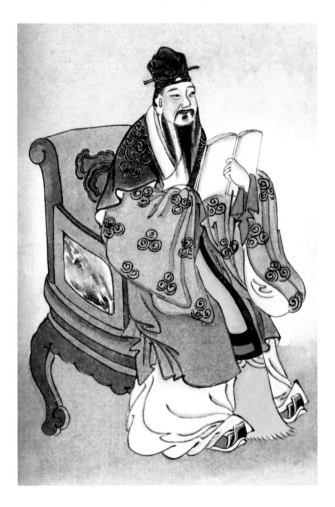

Right The philosopher Mencius.

Unknown Unknowns

The Chinese texts discussed here are not referred to in any other Tai Chi books I know of. They are nonetheless very important for Tai Chi practitioners, as they explore key ideas around Nei Dan/internal alchemy, martial arts and Qi cultivation, all part of the 'big picture' in Tai Chi.

Nei Ye

Professor Harold D Roth's book *Original Tao – Inward Training and the Foundations of Taoist Mysticism* is a translation of Nei Ye (Inward Training), a collection of poetic verses on the Tao, meditation and breathing, which he dates from the mid-4th century BCE. He uses the title *Original Tao* as 'it represents the earliest extant presentation of a mystical practice that appears in all the earliest sources of Taoist thought'. The text was buried in a work called *Guan Zi* (The Writings of Master Guan), attributed to the famous minister Guan Zhong of the 7th century BCE.

Much of what has survived from this period was passed down by oral tradition; the same is true of The Tai Chi Chuan Classics, and the mnemonic nature of Nei Ye suggests that it too was originally transmitted in this way.

The terminology found in Nei Ye has resonances not only with Laozi and Zhuangzi, but also with The Tai Chi Chuan Classics. The character Zheng crops up again and again – it is often translated by Tai Chi exponents as 'erect', but, as we saw in our discussion of the *Yi Jing*, it really means correctly aligned. The Nei Ye is of unique importance to Tai Chi practitioners because it explains how we should feel before, during and after our practice.

Roth believes that early (non-religious) Taoism consisted 'of a number of closely related master/disciple lineages, all of which followed a common cultivation practice first enunciated in *Inward Training*'. These individual lineages would mainly have been small independent groups and could not be said to be cults or even organized sects. The links between early Taoists and what Roth calls the 'cult of immortality' to which practitioners of physical and macrobiotic hygiene belonged need further examination, as does the influence of both on Tai Chi Chuan and Qigong. However, then as now, such activities were unpopular with the political elite, because to take them seriously meant devoting your life to them and failing in your duty to produce descendants and serve the state.

The wisdom we obtain from Nei Ye includes:

'The Way [Tao] penetrates the limitless [Wu Chi].'

'Cultivate the mind and be of correct form [Zheng Xing]' This concept of attaining the correct body alignment is a recurring theme in Tai Chi.

'For Heaven, the principle is to be correct [Zheng].
For Earth the principle is to be level.
For persons, the principle is to be still.'

So we need to keep our spine/centre line straight and our shoulders level. When we practise Tai Chi, we start from a formal still position.

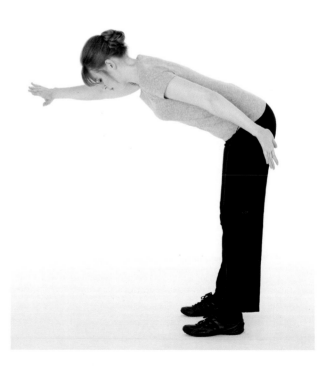

Right White Crane Flaps its Wings: inclined, but centrally correct.

'If you are correct [Zheng] you can be still.
Then you can be balanced [Ding]…'

Zhong Ding/Central Equilibrium is the state we normally want to be in when practising Tai Chi Form, Pushing Hands, weapons or Neigong.

'…With the mind stable and centred,
With ears and eyes listening [Ting] and comprehending…'

Ting is a compound character, representing a disciple ten times using the eyes, the ears and the heart mind to listen.

'…With the four limbs solid and firm
You can then act as a home for the vital essence [Jing].
The vital essence; it is the vital energy [Qi]'s vital essence.
When the vital energy is made to flow, the vital essence is born.'

In Tai Chi terms correct practice leads to calm, stability and awareness and stimulates the respiration and circulation. But according to a well-known tenet of Chinese philosophy, 'Excessive correctness [Zheng] is perversion.'

'When the shape/body isn't correct,
Virtue doesn't come.
When the centre isn't stable,
The mind isn't pure.
With correct shape, virtue will come.'

Whether we are dealing with Tai Chi or meditation, bad posture and bad technique will not only have negative physical effects such as interrupting the breathing and circulation; they will also affect concentration and spirit.

The Nei Ye aims at getting the mind correct:

'A correct mind in the centre,
And the Ten Thousand Things attain their due limit.'

We now know that exercise helps to maintain or even increase bone density. People knew this from their daily practice more than 2,000 years ago:

'If people are able to be correct and stable,
The skin is ample and smooth,
The ears and eyes listen and comprehend.
The sinews are stretched and the bones are strengthened.
Then they'll be able to bear the Big Circle [of Heaven]
And to tread over the Big Square [of Earth].'

Note the duality the author used to refer to things we do every day in Tai Chi practice, such as listen and comprehend:

'All who follow the Way
Must revolve, must close,
Must unwind, must expand,
Must be stable, must be constant.
Attend to doing things well and don't neglect them
Drive out excesses and forsake what is indifferent.
When you can attain the Ultimate Limit [Chi, as in Tai Chi]
Return to the Way and Virtue.'

The Classic of the Way and Virtue is, of course, the title of Laozi's book.

We discussed how Confucius used body language and how good body language was essential in Tai Chi. The book Nei Ye thinks so too. It also talks of the limit/ultimate in vital essence and vital energy (Jing Qi), when the four limbs are correct, while the blood and vital energy are stable. We are of one intent and mind.

In Tai Chi practice we need to maintain concentration and not get side-tracked. Again, the Nei Ye thinks so too:

'Let a balanced and correct breathing fill the chest.
…this brings longevity.'

The author also refers to the Oneness beloved by Laozi (and Tai Chi):

'So we need good Qi and good bodies to get the most out of life.
Let the chest (when breathing) be level and straight
[This sentence is repeated at the end of the chapter. Presumably the author considered it to be important.]
It ripples and blends in the mind.
This results in long life.'

You need to move when you're full or the vital energy won't flow. If you don't forget your troubles when you're old, it'll drain the vital energy.
The Song of the Thirteen Tactics intones,

'Internally the abdomen is relaxed and still
And the Qi ascends.'

The Nei Ye is of like mind:

'Accumulate, then release.'

'When you make your mind big and release it,
When you relax and broaden the vital energy,
And the body is peaceful and doesn't shift,
And you can preserve the One and reject
Ten Thousand inconsequentials.'

The Dalai Lama once remarked that without peace of
mind, it's impossible to meditate. Fortunately regular Tai
Chi practice helps to induce the essential stillness and
equilibrium mentioned by the Nei Ye:

'Supernatural vital energy resides in the heart.
There's one coming and one departing.
Its delicacy is such that there's nothing inside.
Its vastness is such that there's nothing outside.
So we lose it.
Because rashness is harmful
And the mind can maintain stillness,
The Tao will naturally be in equilibrium.
As for folk who've acquired the Tao,
It penetrates the skin and seeps into the hair.
At the centre of the breast there is no defeat.
The Tao of restraining the desires is such
That the Ten Thousand Things can't harm you.'

Heguanzi (c. 5th –2nd century BCE)

The writings of Heguanzi (whose name means Pheasant
Cap Master) were collated at some time during the
Warring States period (475–221 BCE), a time of change,
upheaval and shifting alliances. The text is liberal in
flavour and talks of the Tao, of leadership, strategy,
alchemy, meditation and much more.

The famous Wing Chun master Wong Shun-leung
once said that you have to be very poor or very rich to be
good at martial arts, as otherwise you won't have enough
time to practise:

'The noble have knowledge
The rich have wealth.
The poor have their bodies.'
Heguanzi

It seems that internal alchemy techniques and the concept
of the Three Treasures were popular more than 2,000
years ago:

'Control is how he protects essence
and uplifts spirit to induce energy
He conserves it so it does not leak.'

Tai Chi is sometimes called Shadow Boxing and we are
like our opponent's shadow, moving as he moves.

'Shadow follows form,
echo responds to sound.'

If we are going to use Tai Chi for self-defence we must be
ready to get hurt and to hurt the opponent also:

'The courageous knight does not fear to die
and to obliterate his name.'

An Interpretation of the Practice of the 13 Tactics tells us:

'The Qi sticks to the back;
It amasses and enters the spine.
Internally it strengthens the vigour [Jingshen],
Externally we exhibit peaceful ease.'

As Heguanzi puts it:

'When mind is master,
The internal will command the external.'

The Book of Balance and Harmony

The author of this 13th-century work was Li Daoqun,
a student of 16 or more masters, who is supposed
to have learned 'the final secret' from 'a mysterious
personage' in Central Asia. Though there has been a
veritable plethora of such personages floating around at
various times – and not just in Central Asia – some of the
material is immensely interesting to Tai Chi practitioners.
Furthermore, Li later became a master of the Complete
Reality School of Taoism, to which Tai Chi Chuan
patriarch Zhang Sanfeng has been linked. He also wrote
commentaries on the Tai Chi Diagram of neo-Confucian
philosopher Zhou Dunyi.

The Book of Balance and Harmony is divided into
20 sections covering alchemy, Taoistic practices –
including meditation, breathing and sex – philosophy,
poems, commentaries and criticisms. One of the
alchemical passages is similar to one of 40 texts published
by the great Tai Chi families of Wu and Yang (though
never explained by them) and ascribed to Zhang
Sanfeng. Buddhism, especially of the Chan variety, is
often mentioned. There's a well-established connection
between Chan Buddhism and the Complete Reality
School. In 1984 I saw Taoist imagery, including the Tai
Chi symbol, among the ruins of the (Buddhist) Shaolin
Temple, and Buddhist imagery, including gods and
swastikas, among the (Taoist) temples on Wudang Mountain.

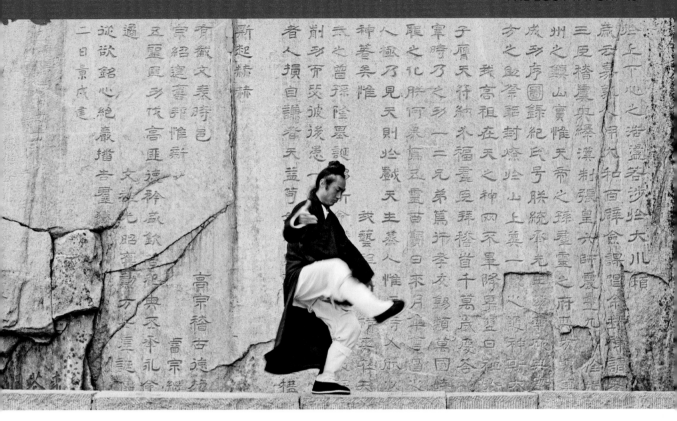

Above A Taoist monk practising Tai Chi.

In Part Seven of *The Book of Balance and Harmony*, 'The Gold-Testing Stone', we find 'Sages, using their power of skilful means [note the use of a Buddhist concept], have opened up good avenues of introduction, setting up terminology and imagery, writing alchemical treatises to guide students.'

Another section covers various grades of practice. The 'Upper Middle Grade' covers the transmission of initiation and precepts, readings and recitation, and thus has parallels with the Bai Shi initiation ritual for disciples used in many Tai Chi schools, including my own.

The 'Lower Upper Grade' mentions meditative breathing, massage, physical exercises, keeping the attention on the navel and swallowing copious amounts of saliva – all part of regular Tai Chi and Qigong practice.

The 'Middle Upper Grade' mentions circulatory methods, bending and stretching and twisting the spine – all Tai Chi methods of practice. The 'Higher Upper Grade' is mainly concerned with internal alchemy.

Part Thirteen, 'Some Questions on Alchemy' has the question, 'Strum the lute to call the phoenix.' What does this mean?

It's a metaphor for emptying the mind and nourishing the spirit. This would seem to explain the frequent appearance of Stroking the Lute/Seven Stars (essentially the same technique) in Yang lineage Long Forms: a major application of this technique is to come to an on-guard position to face a new attack or opponent, thus necessitating 'emptying the mind'.

There are interesting thoughts on spiritual alchemy, including 'When the mind is settled the spirit is complete; when the spirit is complete one perfects essence.' This explains the ritualistic preparatory movements in many Tai Chi schools prior to entering the practice of form or Neigong. There are also passages on movement and stillness and other relevant dualities.

Part Eighteen, 'Songs', contains references to the Northern Dipper and by extension is also a metaphor for the Seven Stars techniques which we have in Tai Chi. 'A mystic pearl' and later 'a tiny pearl' are mentioned and may again be the pearl with nine crooked paths mentioned earlier (see page 23).

There are also many references to Qigong techniques to be found in Immortal Family Baduanjin and to the Tai Chi Neigong technique Embracing the One.

The final section of the book, 'Veiled Words', deals with delusion and fixation and removing 'habit-conditioned energy', which is a prime purpose of internal training. Lastly it talks about knowing how and where to stop.

As you can see, the nay-sayers are right, what they practice truly has little or nothing to do with Taoism. For the rest of us it is clear that Tai Chi is firmly rooted in Taoism (even though there are a few aspects of the art from other sources).

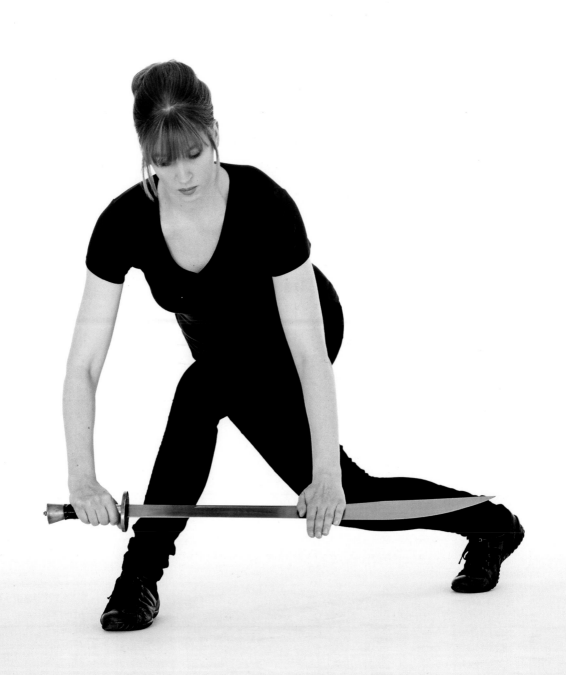

2 The Lost History of Tai Chi – Killer Questions

This chapter is concerned with how Tai Chi gradually emerged from the morass that was Imperial China. We'll also discuss some of the practitioners who developed it. My Sifu called the Chinese martial arts 'the world of truth and lies'. In Tai Chi history there are few truths and many lies, many known unknowns, plenty of unknown unknowns and more than one unknown known. The reader should be aware that in what follows, as always seems to be the case with Tai Chi, known knowns are few and far between.

Tai Chi History Question Time

This unusual approach to a complex subject is the brainchild of, Dr Alex Ryan. For further reading, refer to the Tai Chi Book Group on page 240.

Before Tai Chi Became Public – Out in the Boondocks

Q: What do we know about martial arts in imperial China?

Successive Chinese regimes, both imperial and communist, have attempted to regulate, control, repress and prohibit the practice of Chinese martial arts. The authorities didn't like the idea of private citizens learning how to fight; they saw martial arts teachers as a threat, especially in view of the intense bond of the master/disciple relationship.

Nevertheless, generations of Chinese peasants practised their village boxing to protect their homes against bandits, rival villages and rebellions led by sects such as White Lotus (1796–1804), Eight Trigrams (1813) and the Taiping (Supreme Peace) rebels (1850–64). In the Taiping Rebellion alone, more than 20 million died.

Q: What are the legends around Tai Chi development?

There are three main stories relating to the origins of Tai Chi. They are the Chen family story, the Taoism story and the Nobody Knows option.

The Chen Family Story

It is natural that the martial art of the Chen family village (Chenjiagou) should have been influenced by Shaolin methods, as they are both in Henan province, only a few hours apart by road.

According to the Chens, their first-generation ancestor, Chen Bu, started the martial arts tradition within their village in the late 14th century. Problem: there's no evidence for this claim whatsoever. Furthermore, for many years the Chens claimed that all aspects of Chen family boxing, including Tai Chi Chuan, originated with their clan. It's an unknown known. They want it to be true, but it's not.

According to the same tradition, the ninth-generation Chen patriarch, Chen Wangting (c. 1580–1660), codified Chen family boxing into seven routines. This supposedly included five routines of Tai Chi Chuan, the 108-technique Long Fist Form and a more rigorous routine known as Cannon Punch (Pao Chui). Only one Tai Chi routine and the Pao Chui routine have survived.

In a report dated 9 June 1980 in the *Physical Education Newspaper*, Chen-style teacher and historian Gu Liuxin said that he had formerly confused the Chen Wangting who came from the Chen village and, in 1640, had led rural militia to support the local magistrate against an oppressive warlord, and the Chen Wangting from South Manchuria who had been an Imperial Censor and received awards from the Emperor before his death in 1630. In reality, the Ting characters in the two names are different, so it unlikely that a Chinese scholar would have confused them. There is also an enormous social gulf between an Imperial Censor and a leader of rural militia.

Corroborating Gu's report, Tai Chi historian Wu Tunan wrote of his 1917 visit to the Chen village. He'd met the schoolmaster, Chen Xin, and gone with him to the family graveyard; written on Chen Wangting's tombstone were the words Wu Xiang Sheng, meaning a military graduate at county level, the equivalent to a modern-day elementary/primary school graduate – an average 11 year old. Most Tai Chi historians accept that Chen Wangting was a pivotal character in Chen family martial arts. Note that I don't use the term Tai Chi.

In October 1995 I was taken round the Chen village by Chen Zaosen, a senior Chen-style instructor. I saw that all the old tombstones had been removed from the cemetery and lain on the ground outside the Pao Chui training hall. None of them mentioned Tai Chi Chuan. Bright new tombstones had been erected in the cemetery, praising the Chen family ancestors and their contribution to Tai Chi Chuan. All the new monuments and tombstones honoured Chen Wangting as the founder of Tai Chi Chuan. But I did not see a single item of antiquity which mentioned Tai Chi Chuan.

I asked about the grave of Chen Changxing, the great master who taught Tai Chi Chuan to Yang Luchan, founder of the Yang style. I couldn't see his grave in the cemetery and was told that there wasn't one. Nor is he honoured in the Chen family Pao Chui training hall; apart from his name on a new black tablet in the training hall giving the Chen family martial arts lineage, the only sign of him that I could find in the village was in a museum created with Taiwanese money in the grounds of the house where he taught. I don't believe all this is an accident: it's clear that the Chen family did not approve

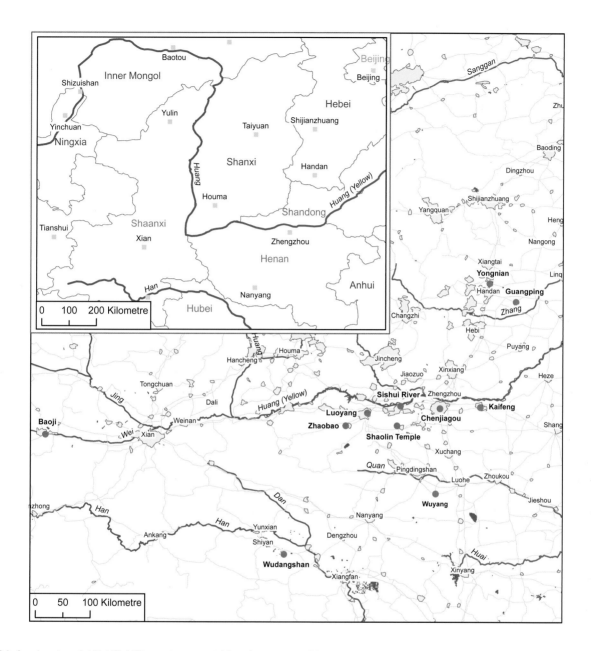

of his having taught Tai Chi Chuan to an outsider. As we psychologists say, there are no accidents.

Above A map showing important Tai Chi locations marked in red. Inset; a general map of the region.

The Taoism Story

The first text hailing Zhang Sanfeng as the creator of Tai Chi was written by Li Yiyu, nephew of Wu Yuxiang, in his *Short Introduction to Tai Chi Chuan* in 1880, although a tradition that Zhang was the founder of Internal Boxing dates back to 1669. Most Tai Chi books of whatever language or era take the position that Zhang was the founder, and though this is based on an oral tradition, that doesn't mean it's wrong. Not everything is written down; not even on Wikipedia. To this day in many Tai

Chi schools, including my own, the ceremony of ritual initiation for disciples identifies him as the founder of Tai Chi – it's a sore point with the Chens.

There is no official record of Zhang before the Ming dynasty (1368–1644). He was first linked with martial arts in a tombstone inscription of 1669, but this referred to him in connection with Internal Family Boxing (see Glossary on page 230); Tai Chi isn't mentioned.

German Sinologist and expert on Taoism Anna Seidel wrote of him, 'He was a Taoist master loosely connected with the local centre of the Quanzhen (Complete Reality) sect on Wudang Mountain and he was very famous in the Hongwu and Yongle eras (1368–1424) since he attracted the attention of these two emperors. He continued to act upon the imagination of amateurs of the miraculous in the following centuries, to the point of being canonized and wrapped in a wreath of legends.'

The Nobody Knows Option

Li Yiyu wrote in his introduction to The Tai Chi Chuan Classics, 'The founder of Tai Chi is unknown.'

Q: What do we know about Nei Jia Chuan/ Internal Family Boxing and how does it connect with Tai Chi?

Tai Chi is sometimes referred to as Nei Jia Chuan/Internal Family Boxing because certain aspects of the art are taught only after ritual initiation; because of the emphasis on the intent and spirit; and because of its connection with Nei Dan/internal alchemy.

The earliest, definite, historical reference to what seems to have been an internal Chinese martial art is the story of the poet, scholar and martial artist Chen Yuanbin. We know that in 1621 he visited Japan. Around 1638, to escape the then rising Manchu Qing dynasty in China, he settled in Nagasaki and secured a position with the nobles of the Owariha family. During this time he produced many treatises and texts on Chinese philosophy and was responsible for introducing the works of many Chinese poets into the mainstream of Japanese culture.

Chen also taught three Ronin (masterless samurai) his Chinese boxing method. This was later called Jujutsu, meaning soft technique and suggesting an art similar in approach to Tai Chi, where softness is used to overcome hardness.

In 1649 scholar, statesman, Ming patriot and martial artist Huang Zongxi (1610–95) and other resistance leaders went to Nagasaki to seek help against the Manchus. Given their backgrounds and the Nagasaki connection it seems likely that Chen Yuanbin and Huang were acquainted.

Huang's internal martial arts master was Wang Zhengnan, and in 1669 Huang inscribed this epitaph on his master's tombstone: 'Shaolin boxing is famous in the world and concentrates on attacking the opponent's weak points. People can therefore take advantage of this. In the so-called Nei Jia (Internal Family), stillness is used to control movement: when the opponent attacks, then he is countered. So Shaolin is called Wai Jia (External Family). The origins [of Nei Jia] are mainly from Zhang Sanfeng. Sanfeng was a Wudang Taoist. The Emperor Hui Zong (1101–25) sent for him, but though he arrived, he did not succeed in meeting the Emperor. In a dream Zhang was

taught boxing by the Emperor Xuan Di and the next day he killed more than a hundred bandits.'

The Zhang Sanfeng who is regarded as the founder of Tai Chi lived around the mid-14th century till the early 15th, so either there were two Zhang Sanfengs living at different periods or the dates given here are wrong.

Huang was a committed Confucian who practised Jingzuo (quiet sitting meditation). He was also reputed to be expert in Dim Mak (attacking pressure points). In 1676, his son, Huang Baijia, compiled the first Internal Family Boxing manual.

We can deduce from all this that in the mid-17th century something similar to Tai Chi in combat approach was being practised.

When Tai Chi Appeared

Q: Where do we first see something recognizable as Tai Chi?

The first person we know of who taught something that we might recognize as Tai Chi was Yang Luchan (1799–1872). He brought the art to Beijing in 1852. This seems to have been when the term Tai Chi Chuan was first used. Having learned Tai Chi in the remote Chen village, probably with very little contact with practitioners of other systems, Yang may have come across influences in Beijing that caused him to alter his approach considerably.

It was a long way from the Chen village to Beijing – in more ways than one.

Q: How did the different Tai Chi styles evolve?

A convenient truth is that all the authentic Tai Chi practised today is ultimately mainly Chen lineage or mainly Yang lineage in origin. But what do we mean by lineage?

I've always liked the mavericks, people who think for themselves. My Sifu was like that; I try to be like that. Despite all I've said and all I'm going to say, whether inside or outside the family, there are only two kinds of Tai Chi tutor, good ones and bad ones. But Tai Chi isn't a museum piece; sometimes changes are necessary.

The Chinese use five main terms to denote a style of martial arts. The first and most obvious one is Chuan, which literally means fist, as in Tai Chi Chuan/Supreme Ultimate Fist; this is the general term for all the family and non-family Tai Chi styles.

The next term in common use is Jia or family, as in Wu Jia or Wu family. There is a real problem here. Members of the famous Tai Chi families like to give the impression that the art has been passed down through the family unchanged from generation to generation. This is not true: of course it has evolved over time.

The third term is Shi, which means work done after a model or pattern; in a Tai Chi context it is often taken to mean lineage. So for example Wu Shi means in the model/lineage of Wu – but which Wu? My Sifu considered that, while we were part of the Wu lineage, we also had other influences in our own version of Tai Chi.

The fourth term is Men, meaning door or gate. Those 'inside the door' are disciples of the style. All others are outsiders. When I saw my old blind and crippled Sifu for the last time, he told me he'd left the Wudang gate – he no longer considered himself an insider.

Finally, the term Pai means school or sect. It is often used in connection with schools of philosophy or religious sects, but also with reference to schools of Tai Chi such as Hao Pai/Hao school.

For a style to be called Tai Chi Chuan it is not enough that it contains slow and relaxed movements. I could teach Karate or Wing Chun in this way with no difficulty; some people actually do this very thing. But to earn the name Tai Chi Chuan there must be a lineage, a clear connection between what is being practised and The Tai Chi Chuan Classics.

Q: What is the link between Tai Chi and *The Classic of Boxing*?

For many years the Chens claimed that all aspects of Chen family boxing, including Tai Chi Chuan, originated with the Chen clan. The simple but inconvenient truth for the Chens (who until recent times claimed to be practicing a pure family art) is that the Chen family Hand Forms contain the names of 29 of the 32 techniques found in *The Classic of Boxing*. Written by the Ming General Qi Jiguang (1528–87), *The Classic of Boxing* is said to represent a synthesis of 16 different schools of boxing. The Chens now say Chen Wangting introduced the 29 techniques to Chen boxing.

In the Yang lineage (see page 248), the names of at most eight techniques come from *The Classic of Boxing*. If we compare techniques of the same name from Tai Chi and from *The Classic of Boxing*, we find that the applications, strangely, are almost uniformly different. In *The Classic of Boxing* there is some mention of the concepts of softness and evasion, but the vast majority of techniques are applied differently from Yang lineage techniques.

For example, the drawing of the second technique of *The Classic of Boxing*, Golden Cockerel Stands on One Leg, bears a strong resemblance to the Tai Chi technique of the same name, though the application described in the accompanying ditty is nothing like any of the regular Tai Chi applications of this technique. To make matters clearer see the table in Appendix I (see page 233) of

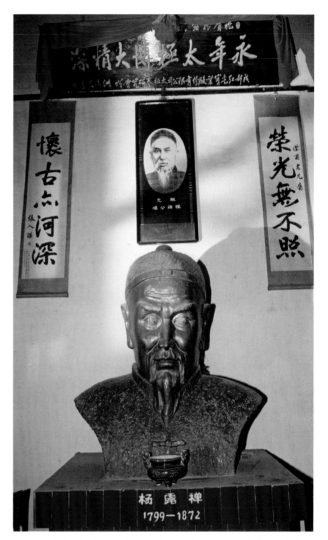

Above A bust of Chen Changxing and above it a picture of his student, Yang Luchan in the Chen village.

The Classic of Boxing techniques and the appearance of eight of them in Yang lineage Long Forms.

The Chens suggest that the Yangs changed the Chen old-style Tai Chi Chuan and Pao Chui forms which Chen Changxing taught them (Tai Chi historian Gu Liuxin suggests it was Yang Luchan's sons). But there is no evidence for this and there is a host of other differences anyway.

If Yang lineage techniques come from the Chen family art, why do only some have a connection with *The Classic of Boxing*, and why are none of the inner techniques of the Yang lineage Long Forms, or the techniques of the Tai Chi Neigong or Pushing Hands mentioned in *The Classic of Boxing*? Most of the techniques therein don't resemble Yang lineage techniques, either in their names or in the illustrations or descriptions given. So the names of techniques might have been borrowed from *The Classic of Boxing* and applied to quite different Tai Chi techniques.

So there are links between Tai Chi and *The Classic of Boxing*, but they are not clear cut.

Q: What do we know about Yang Luchan teaching in Guangping?

According to Yang Luchan's illustrated story, which I read at the Yang family museum in 1997, he made three trips from Guangping to the Chen village for Tai Chi study. We don't know how long he spent there on each visit, nor do we know the length of time between each visit.

At some point, most likely after his initial sojourn in the Chen village, he returned to Guangping, made a connection with Wu Yuxiang (1812–80) and his two brothers, and began to teach them Tai Chi. The two brothers held official positions and the Wu family were wealthy landlords who belonged to the cultural elite. This family has never been renowned in Tai Chi circles as fighters and it is likely that the training Yang Luchan gave them reflected that.

Given Yang's later reputation, I would guess that teaching the gentry bored him rigid.

Q: Who were Yang's key students and what were their legacies?

Yang Luchan's most significant students before he moved to Beijing were the Wu brothers, in particular Wu Yuxiang. Without their help, he'd probably never have had the chance to teach in the Forbidden City and Tai Chi might have disappeared into obscurity. The Wu brothers were interesting characters. They were members of the literati; they wrote about Tai Chi theory; they came from Yang Luchan's home town of Guangping; they gave him the connection to Beijing.

Wu Yuxiang's nephew, Li Yiyu, tells us how his uncle visited Zhaobao in 1852, en route from Guangping to the Chen village. This is unlikely; it is over 500km (300 miles) from Guangping to the town of Zhaobao, and by no stretch of the imagination is it on the way to the Chen village. Another Tai Chi historical lie.

Wu Yuxiang is supposed to have trained in Zhaobao under Chen Qingping (1795–1868) for one month and to have learned all his secrets. After this he made the Tai Chi of Zhaobao, a variation on the Chen style, known outside the area; it led him to develop his own style, which in turn produced the Hao and Sun styles.

In addition to teaching the Wus, Yang Luchan had two sons, Yang Banhou and Yang Jianhou, who also became famous Tai Chi masters. Yang Banhou is reputed to have been much more aggressive than his brother. Being the elder, he was his father's main assistant and is said to have been bested by a couple of senior students, Wang Lanting and Chen Xiufeng. When teaching Manchu princes in the Forbidden City, Yang Luchan personally put them through the Bai Shi ceremony of discipleship. Lesser mortals went through the ceremony with one of his sons, as they couldn't be seen to be on the same level as members of the royal family.

Yang Banhou's most accomplished student was Wu Quanyou (no relation – the Chinese character for his surname is different from that of Wu Yuxiang). He was known for his skills in neutralizing and evasion and is considered to be the founder of the other Wu style of Tai Chi. The ethnic Chinese court official Wang Lanting was also very effective and, it is said, had to seek sanctuary after killing some Manchus.

For a complete translation and analysis of *The Classic of Boxing*, please see my book *Tai Chi Chuan – Decoding the Classics for the Modern Martial Artist*. For a comparison of *The Classic of Boxing* techniques with Yang lineage techniques of the same name, see my book *The Tai Chi Bible*.

Q: Where could the differences between the Yang lineage and Chen lineage have come from?

There are a number of possibilities. One is that Yang Luchan blended skills from other arts with what he had learned from Chen Changxing. If this happened it was probably in Beijing, when he was meeting the top men in other systems.

More likely is that most of these techniques had another origin – that, as the Yang-lineage schools maintain, Tai Chi was brought to the Chen village from outside by Jiang Fa, who was a student of Wang Zongyue, a teacher and scholar resident in Kaifeng in 1791 and in Luoyang in 1795. These cities are quite close to the Chen village.

This could be why Yang's teacher, Chen Changxing, is not honoured by the Chen family, having chosen an outsider as his master and forsaken the Chen tradition of Pao Chui for Tai Chi.

The Chens maintain that Wang Zongyue was a contemporary of their clan's 13th generation. If so, he could have taught Jiang Fa and even Chen Changxing. Chen historians such as Tang Hao, have suggested that Wang learned his art from the Chen clan; there is no evidence for this claim.

The Chen material is not clear about who, if anyone, learned from Wang and Jiang; according to them all lines of transmission of the Chen art are through Chen clansmen until the time of Yang Luchan. However, there is evidence from Tang Hao, writing in the 1940s and '50s, that Chen Xin tried to suppress rumours among Chen villagers that Jiang Fa taught Chen Changxing.

Q: Did Chen Changxing learn Tai Chi Chuan from another member of the Chen clan or from an outsider?

Yang Luchan died in 1872. We don't know every detail about the form or forms which he taught, but we can compare forms taught by those who follow him in the lineage. Admittedly there are a few variations in the sequence, and sometimes slightly different names are used for the same techniques in the Long Forms practised by my school, the Wu Jianquan school, and others such as the Yang Chengfu and Wu Yuxiang schools. But the sequence itself and the names of the techniques are largely uniform. The way of moving is similar, too: continuous, smooth and slow.

The Chens claim that Chen Changxing taught the 'old two Tao Lu (forms) in Big Frame' and that this is what was handed down by his great-grandson Chen Fake (1887–1957) to the present generation. I believe that historian Wu Tunan was right and that before Jiang Fa brought Tai Chi to the village, Chen Changxing taught orthodox Chen family boxing. After instruction from Jiang Fa, he blended his new Tai Chi knowledge with some of the Chen family techniques to produce a hybrid which he taught to Yang and others. This did not make him popular with the Chen clan.

Tai Chi and the Qing Empire

Q: Whom did Yang teach and what did he teach them?

The connections Yang Luchan made in Beijing were good ones. Soon after his arrival he had no fewer than eight Manchu princes as his students. His elder son, Yang Banhou, was instructor to the Western Garrison. He and his sons often stayed with Prince Duan (1856–1922), which suggests the prince was one of his students. Duan was a close ally of the Empress Dowager, a significant figure in the imperial court, and later became a national hero for his anti-foreigner stance during the Boxer Rebellion of 1898–1900.

Based on my police riot drill experiences, I surmise that the garrison soldiers were drilled in weapon and hand-to-hand combat en masse, while the princelings and a few favoured bannermen were taught the finer points of the art, including Neigong and internal alchemy, in small 'inside the door' groups. As the Yangs' top student was generally acknowledged to be the Manchu bannerman Wu Quanyou, this would explain the survival

in the Wu family of the 24-exercise Tai Chi Neigong and the heavy internal-alchemy bent of three of the 40 texts given to them by Yang Banhou. It may be that Yang Luchan changed his approach during his two decades in the Forbidden City.

It would be interesting to compare the Yang family syllabus when they were teaching the Wu brothers back in Guangping with what they were teaching in the Forbidden City 20 years later. It should be noted that, of Yang's students, only the Wu brothers are known to have written anything on Tai Chi. Most of his other well-known students were famous as fighters.

Among Yang's disciples, only Yang's sons, the Wu brothers, Wu Quanyou and Wang Lanting went on to become major teachers.

Q: Who else was operating at the time?

Around 1864, Baguazhang/Eight Trigrams Palm adept Dong Haichuan – like Yang Luchan from Hebei province – entered the Forbidden City and joined the household of Prince Su as a servant. After some years, his martial abilities became known and he was given a job teaching martial arts. From this time on Bagua masters were employed as the imperial bodyguards. Bagua emphasizes evasion, footwork and turning.

At around the same time, Guo Yunshen, yet another man from Hebei province, was employed to teach Xingyi (Form and Intent) Boxing at Duke Yu's residence. This is a very different martial art from Tai Chi: Xingyi emphasizes direct impact. Tai Chi is by turns evasive and direct.

Q: How favoured was Tai Chi/where does it fit in this climate?

Perhaps partly because he had two sons to help him, perhaps because of his high level of skill, Yang seems to have been more successful and more active than his fellow internal martial artists.

Q: What was the context around Tai Chi's move into the centre of power?

Once we start dealing with the Forbidden City, Tai Chi history becomes much more interesting and much more complex.

Built between 1406 and 1420 in the heart of Beijing, the palace complex of the Forbidden City (the largest in the world) was an imperial palace for almost 500 years. It was called the Forbidden City because entrance was forbidden to anyone who did not have imperial authority to visit. With the abdication of the last emperor, Puyi, in 1912, the Forbidden City ceased to be the centre of the Chinese universe.

As we have seen, it is generally agreed that Yang Luchan brought Tai Chi to the Forbidden City in 1852, during the Qing dynasty. The Qing were ethnically Manchurian (hence their alternative name of the Manchu dynasty) and hundreds of thousands of Manchu, Chinese and Mongolian troops were stationed in and around the Forbidden City. At that time, China was in the throes of the Taiping Rebellion. The country was ruled by the weak Emperor Xianfeng (ruled 1851–61) who died young and was succeeded by his six-year-old son, Tongzhi. The boy's diminutive mother became Empress Dowager Cixi.

Tongzhi was a bisexual who began visiting Beijing brothels incognito at the age of 15; unsurprisingly he contracted a sexually transmitted disease. His heavy drinking damaged his health still more. The Empress Dowager was the subject of a number of scandals involving young officers and supposed eunuchs whom she promoted for services rendered.

I've visited the Forbidden City many times and its immensity is immediately obvious. It measures 960 x 750m (3,150 x 2,460ft); there are around 800 buildings containing more than 8,700 rooms. At one time during the Ming dynasty period (1368–1644),

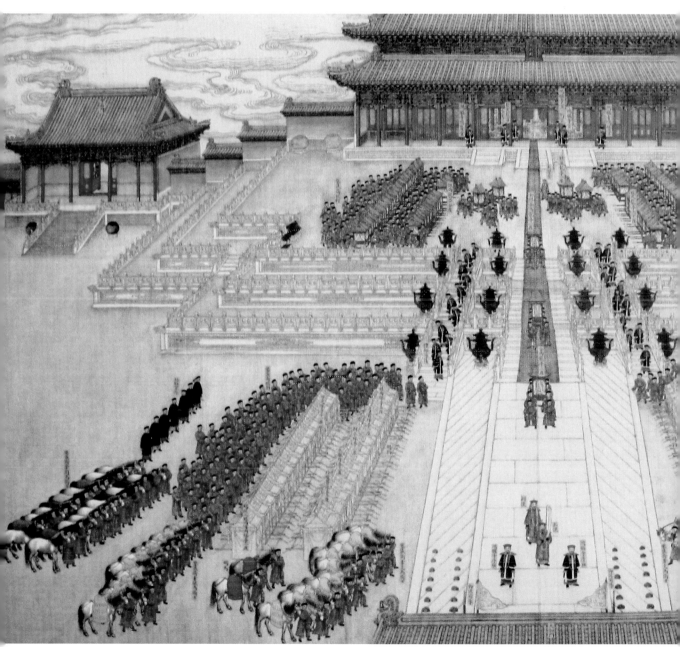

these rooms housed more than 10,000 eunuchs, though by the early 20th century the number was down to around 1,000.

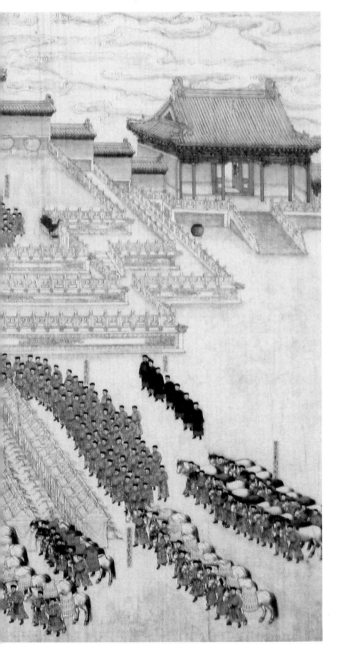

Aftermath – Empire Sundown and Tai Chi for the Masses

Q: Who was responsible for popularizing Tai Chi in China?

Yang Luchan's younger son, Yang Jianhou, was popular and easy-going and had many students. His own son, Yang Chengfu, was a similar personality; he travelled the length and breadth of China, teaching Tai Chi and producing new teachers from among his disciples.

Wu Quanyou's descendants were more organized than the Yangs and every bit as well-connected politically.

Yang Chengfu, Wu Jianquan (see page 66) and their sons became itinerant teachers, travelling constantly to pass on the art, while Sun Lutang, of whom we shall hear more later, wrote about Tai Chi, identifying it as an internal martial art for the first time. This active approach gave Tai Chi critical mass.

Q: What changed as it became available to the masses?

Only the rich could afford to train with the top tutors; to please them the art was simplified and much of the martial content was not passed on. The emphasis was on health and well-being. Later Tai Chi was taught in the Jing Wu (health and martial arts gyms) which sprang up in large cities; classes there were more active. Jing Wu rejected Bai Shi/ritual initiation, so aspects of Tai Chi connected with this, such as Neigong, fell out of favour.

More and more Tai Chi instructors appeared and the laws of supply and demand came into play. Now there are more Tai Chi tutors and practitioners than ever, but the percentage of high-quality tutors hasn't increased. Unfortunately most students will go to the nearest or the cheapest tutor.

Q: What happened to Tai Chi during the Cultural Revolution?

I've spoken to a number of Chinese masters on this. They told me some masters were arrested and beaten, access to normal halls and open practice areas was banned and some famous masters such as Wu Kungcho and Wang Peisheng were sent to Laogai (Reform through Labour) work camps for many years of brutal slavery.

Left A military parade in the Forbidden City.

Historical Snapshot

Zhang Sanfeng and Nei Jia Chuan

Tai Chi historian Wu Tunan (1884–1989) acquired a faded copy of *Song Style Family Tai Chi Gong (Skills) Source and History Clan Analects* around 1908–9. Shortly after this, Song Shuming, secretary to General Yuan Shikai, came to Beijing. He produced a copy of the same book which Wu Tunan had been given, except that Song's copy was entitled *Song Yuan-qiao Tai Chi Gong Source and History Clan Analects*; Song claimed that his ancestor Yuanqiao had written it after learning Tai Chi from Zhang Sanfeng.

In the book Song Yuanqiao claims that he went with six others, including Zhang Songxi, to meet a Master Li on Wudang Mountain. They failed to find Li, but met Zhang Sanfeng at the Temple of the Jade Void (the temple is still there; I've visited it a number of times). Zhang was the master of two of the band of seven, Zhang Songxi and Zhang Cuishan, and from that time on the seven visited Wudang annually to train in Tai Chi with Zhang.

The Master Li they were supposedly searching for was Li Daozi of the Tang dynasty (618–958 CE), who passed on Xian Tian Chuan/Before Heaven Boxing to members of the Yu clan, including Yu Chingwei (one of two men

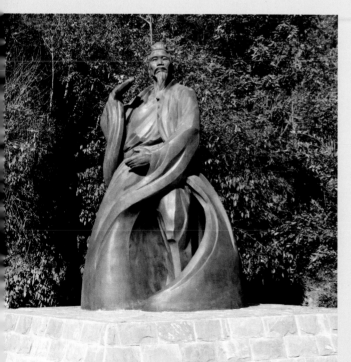

among the seven with the surname of Yu). Li Daozi was also known as Li Daoshan (Li of the Mountain of the Way), perhaps because he lived in the Southern Cliff Palace (it is still there, too) on Wudang Mountain.

Sang's book said that during the time of the Liang dynasty (502–557 CE), Prefect Cheng Lingxi from Anhui province practised Tai Chi Chuan. The art was taught to troops and for several generations within Cheng's family. His descendant, Cheng Mi, a scholar and expert on *Yi Jing*, claimed that his ancestor Lingxi was taught Tai Chi Chuan by Han Gongyue and that the art had existed long before this. Lingxi added elbow techniques and named the art Xiao Jiu Tian/Little Nine Heavens, referring to the Eight Directions and the centre (the Eight Trigrams with the Tai Chi symbol in the centre). A martial method with this name and Taoist origins is still practised in northeast China.

Song's book also said that a giant, hirsute Taoist recluse named Xu Xuanping resided in Xi Zhou at Zi Yang Mountain and taught a Tai Chi Chuan method called San Shi Qi Shi. This is normally translated as 37 Styles, though some give the name as Three Generations Seven, which sounds the same in Chinese. It's also known as Long Boxing.

Xu is mentioned in *Zhang Sanfeng Cheng Liu/Zhang Sanfeng Inheritance*, part of the body of writings which Wu Jianquan's sons claim were given to their family by Yang Banhou. The text purports to have been written by Zhang Sanfeng and mentions Xu as having passed the art down. If Banhou gave the Wus this text it must have been before his death in 1892, in which case it pre-dates Wu Tunan's discovery of the Song book and corroborates it.

Finally, After Heaven Boxing was taught by Yin Lixiang to Hu Jingzi and Song-Zhongshu. Little is known of Yin or his art.

These arts all use Taoist names, and at least three of them are supposed to have been practised during the Tang dynasty, all in the vicinity of Wudang Mountain and Anhui. Though a number of the people mentioned in the lineages of these arts are historical figures, there is no evidence of their involvement with martial arts in general or with Tai Chi in particular, except for what is written in Song's book. But if it is all made up, why aren't more famous founders claimed for these arts?

Left Stautue of Zhang Sanfeng.

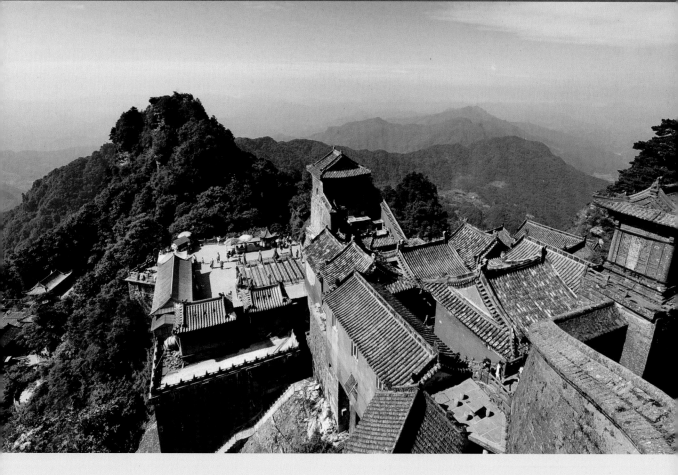

Above View from Golden Peak, Wudang Mountain.

Song's book corroborates *The Biography of Zhang Sanfeng*, attributed to Lu Xixing, in its claim that Zhang Sanfeng learned Tai Chi Chuan on Huashan from a Taoist known as Huo Long/Fire Dragon, though according to Wu Tunan his real name was Jia Desheng. Zhang Sanfeng was supposedly already in his sixties when learning from Huo Long.

Huo Long was taught by Chen Xiyi, a philosopher contemporary to Chu Xi (1130–1200) and a descendant of Chen Tuan. Chen Tuan is credited with developing the Tai Chi Diagram and the Before Heaven Diagram; he also lived on Wudang Mountain as well as on Huashan. Let's analyse all this.

Firstly, if Huo Long learned from a contemporary of Chu Xi, then this would at the latest have been at the end of the 12th century. And if, as the book states, he then taught Zhang Sanfeng, this would have been at the latest in the mid-13th century. Yet we have seen that Zhang was active in the mid-14th and early 15th centuries. The dates don't match. I don't believe that Zhang started to learn Tai Chi at 60 and went on to live for well over 200 years.

As for Zhang Sanfeng being visited by Zhang Songxi and the others, this is at variance with what Wang Weishen has said in *Wudang Zhang Sanfeng Bei Jia Chuan*. Wang has Zhang Songxi living from about 1506 until 1620 and learning the art from Chen Zhoutong, who in turn learned from Wang Zong. This tallies with the fact that Zhang Songxi's grand-student, Wang Zhengnan, died (as we have seen from the tombstone inscription) in 1669. Yet Song's book has Zhang Songxi going to Wudang Mountain and learning from Zhang Sanfeng about 200 years before this. These dates don't match either.

Song Shuming's book gives us some clues about how Tai Chi Chuan may have developed in and from a Taoist philosophical context. Perhaps it explains why the name Tai Chi Chuan was adopted, and the reason behind the quotations from the philosophers Chen Tuan and Zhou Dunyi in The Tai Chi Chuan Classics. Taoism has a history of well over 2,000 years, as do internal alchemy and Chinese martial arts; for these elements to have come together by the time of the Liang or Tang dynasty would hardly be surprising. But remember, it's the world of truth and lies.

Historical Snapshot

The Eclectic Boxer

Before anyone knew what Tai Chi Chuan was, before The Tai Chi Chuan Classics were discovered, somebody else was on the scene.

Chang Naizhou (1724–83) was an eclectic boxer living in Sishui county, Henan province, between Shaolin Temple and the Chen village. Sishui is about 16km (10 miles) from Chen village on the map, but by road it is a tortuous journey of more than 50km (30 miles), as it is necessary to cross the Yellow River. Chang supposedly took up martial arts because he suffered from spontaneous ejaculation.

Chang's writings show an obsession with internal alchemy, acupoints and Qi circulation and cultivation. He even talks about martial application from a Qi perspective. The writings also contain many phrases, sayings and theories found in The Tai Chi Chuan Classics. The question is, did he influence the writing of The Tai Chi Chuan Classics or did The Tai Chi Chuan Classics influence him? The postures and techniques shown in Chang's manual and which I saw performed by Master Liu Yiming as recently as 2007 are very different from those found in any style of Tai Chi.

However, Chang's techniques White Swan (Crane in Tai Chi) Displays Wings and Twin Peaks (Winds in Yang lineage) have similar names to their equivalents in Tai Chi. Another six have the same name as Tai Chi techniques and are to be found in *The Classic of Boxing*. They are Golden Cockerel on One Leg, Seven Stars, Ride the Tiger, Single Whip, Bend the Bow and Tiger Embraces Head. There are also a few techniques that look similar to Tai Chi techniques; for example, Crab Closes Pincers is like Tai Chi's Box the Ears.

Despite Chang's living so close to Chen village, except for a short passage in *The Fighter's Song*, the Chens do not subscribe to The Tai Chi Chuan Classics. However, their main theoretician, Chen Xin, like Chang was into acupoints. It is not known if he also suffered from spermatorrhoea.

Chang's work quotes from *The Classic of Boxing*. Its author, General Qi Jiguang, was an active leader whose men had to be good in armed and unarmed combat as he often sent out five-man patrols to reconnoitre and ambush. Furthermore, Chinese martial arts possess core techniques such as Single Whip, which exist in one form or another in a number of systems such as Long Boxing, as well as in *The Classic of Boxing*.

There are problems with making comparisons of techniques based on the single illustration and short ditty that accompany the name of each technique in *The Classic of Boxing*. Chang himself had the concept of eight phases of how to do techniques, but we don't currently have illustrations to go with this.

Dr Marnix Wells is the only Westerner I know who has trained in this system in Sishui, Chang's birthplace. While there, he interviewed family members who showed him old family manuals and demonstrated their art. Their forms were performed quite fast with coiling and pronounced Fa Jin/Discharge of Skilled Force; they also had techniques mirroring traditional Tai Chi moves such as Double Winds (also known as Box Ears). Unlike most Yang lineage writings, Chang's material actually explains how to use the techniques. The Chang postures, though usually straight, are often in Tai Chi terms somewhat contorted, usually for reasons of application.

Marnix feels straightness can be over-emphasized, as witnessed by those sorry individuals who try to be erect at all times, whether Pushing Hands or fighting. He himself doesn't care for contorted postures, but does not wish to be judgemental and leaves it to the readers to make up their own minds. As a side issue, Chang does mention Central Energy (Qi) and moral rectitude. Another technical difference with 'traditional' Yang Tai Chi is that Chang's boxing sinks onto the tiptoes rather than down into the heels, which Marnix feels may be more effective in promoting mobility.

In terms of source material, Marnix wisely has his doubts about some of the writings of Tang Hao (a solid Chinese Communist and Chen family apologist), though he's more trusting of Xu Zhen, whose examination of the Chen family archives in the 1930s revealed no mention of the term Tai Chi Chuan.

Marnix was unable to ascertain where Chang got hold of the material that is also to be found in the Tai Chi Classics, though there are considerable differences between his boxing and Tai Chi Chuan. Although the principal influence on Chang's writings seems to have been Buddhist, there are elements of Confucianism and to some extent Taoism. Marnix feels the Chang material has been neglected since Xu Zhen looked at it, largely because it falls foul of establishment views of Tai Chi history. Indeed, after the 1930s, Xu Zhen went quiet and there are sound political reasons why.

Marnix and I discussed Yang Luchan's alleged illiteracy and agreed that, like many untutored Chinese, he probably had a good knowledge of how to read and write characters, but not sufficient to write anything as literate as The Tai Chi Chuan Classics. Marnix floated the theory that Wu Yuxiang acquired the books either at the Chen village or at Zhaobao, but there is no evidence for this. Having seen Chang's boxing and read his texts, what I wanted to know was whether or not he cured himself of spermatorrhoea?

Historical Snapshot

Li Yiyu's Preface to The Tai Chi Chuan Classics

An often asked question is where did The Tai Chi Chuan Classics come from? As usual with Tai Chi, it's a known unknown, but there are some stories...

The preface to The Tai Chi Chuan Classics was purportedly written by Wu Yuxiang's nephew Li Yiyu in 1881. Li relates how Wu Yuxiang's brother, Wu Chengqing, on taking up the post of magistrate of Wuyang county, acquired The Tai Chi Chuan Classics in 1852 after they were discovered in a salt cellar. However, the estimable American Tai Chi writer Barbara Davis has shown that this was impossible, as Wu didn't take up his post till 1854. Looking at our map (see page 49), we can see that Wuyang is 430km (270 miles) southwest of Guangping, a long way from where the Tai Chi action was. Apart from Li's discredited story there is no known Tai Chi connection to Wuyang.

Li also asserts that Wang Zongyue (in The Tai Chi Chuan Classics) gives a full explanation of Tai Chi's skills. Li tells us little about Wang, though Tai Chi historians Tang Hao and Xu Yusheng accept him as an active master in the areas of Luoyang and Kaifeng between 1791 and 1795. This view is supported only by an anonymous document, 'Preface to the Manual of the Yinfu Spear', provided by Tang Hao. Given the dates and locations, it's possible that Wang and Chang Naizhou were connected in some way.

Again according to Li Yiyu, Tai Chi was handed down to the Chens of Chen village, who were smart and understood it, but they didn't teach many people. Li tells us little about how the Chens got Tai Chi. They claim to be the true source of the art, yet they accept that the outsider, Wang Zongyue, wrote The Tai Chi Chuan Classics. Many books on Chen Tai Chi include them. Furthermore, while the Classics are respected by all, the Yang lineage puts little or no importance on any writings from the Chens.

A person whom Li describes as 'a certain Yang from our Nanguan township' studied Tai Chi determinedly for more than ten years and reached a high level. After returning home, he taught those who were interested. Li doesn't say it, but 'a certain Yang' can only be an out-of-favour Yang Luchan.

Li's maternal uncle, Wu Yuxiang, liked Tai Chi as soon as he saw it, but Yang wasn't willing to show it, so Wu only got the gist of it. It happens; maybe their karma wasn't right.

Li says it was rumoured that in Zhaobao town, Chen Qingping of the Chen family was skilled in the art. Li gives no details. Chen Qingping is believed by one and all to have learned Chen style while living in the Chen village. Some believe Zhaobao to be a softer variation of Chen style with less emphasis on striking and more on Pushing Hands using locks and trips.

Zhaobao now claims that its Tai Chi comes from Zhang Sanfeng and Wudang Mountain through the usual bunch of mysterious and anonymous Taoists to Wang Zongyue via his student, Jiang Fa, to Zhaobao. There is no evidence whatsoever for this Zhaobao/Zhang Sanfeng connection.

Li claims that in 1852, while on business in Henan, Wu went to Zhaobao and spent more than a month training with Chen Qingping, learning all the special skills. Li gives no details of said skills. Given the facts and the tone of Li's writings, the only logical conclusion to be drawn is that student (Wu) became unhappy with tutor (Yang) and sought out a new tutor (Chen Qingping).

In 1853 Li started to learn Tai Chi from his uncle; despite 20 years training, Li claimed he was only scratching the surface. So he wrote the *Five-Word Formula* to remind himself what he had learned.

So Li Yiyu lied about/was mistaken about the discovery of The Tai Chi Chuan Classics in a salt cellar in 1852. Li also lied about/was mistaken about the circumstances of Wu Yuxiang's trip to Zhaobao.

The strange absence of the Classics from the Chen clan, except for a few phrases, is often discussed and the obvious explanation is that Tai Chi didn't originate with them. The Classics are designed to be chanted, so even if there's no written record, you'd expect them to survive as an oral tradition among practitioners. This is how my Sifu learned them; there's no such tradition among the Chens, though nobody doubts that Chen Changxing taught Tai Chi in the Chen village for a long time.

So what are we to make of Li's preface to The Tai Chi Chuan Classics?

Li had conflicting loyalties as his uncle had later trained in Zhaobao, probably after a falling out with Yang Luchan. Family comes first in China; family comes way before the truth.

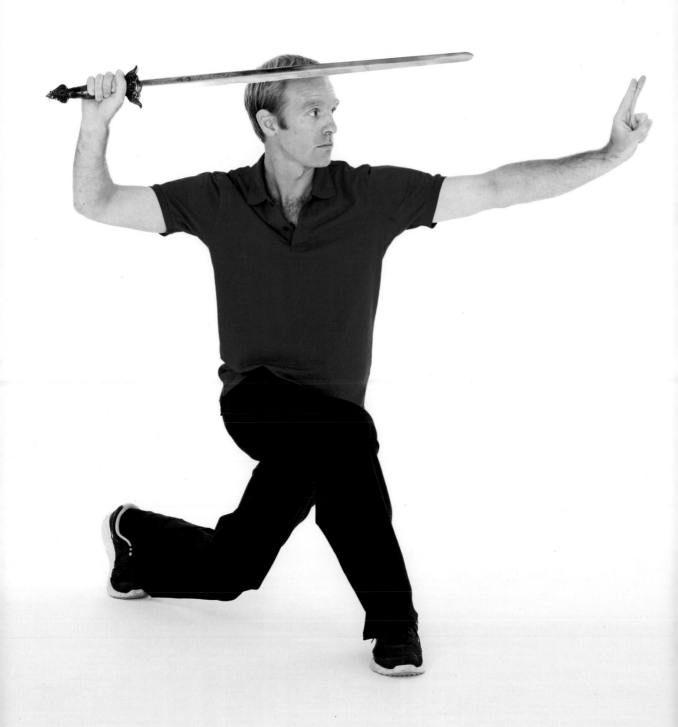

3 Tai Chi Styles

So how do styles come about and why are there so many Tai Chi styles? The short answer is that styles come about because people change things. If we look at photos of Yang Chengfu and Wu Jianquan doing Hand Form, we can clearly see that some techniques are almost identical, while others are quite different. People only began referring to Wu family/style Tai Chi and Yang family/style Tai Chi when they noticed these technical differences between the two. Many Tai Chi authors talk about the five famous Tai Chi families: Chen, Yang, Wu Jianquan, Wu Yuxiang and Sun. Let's look at the various styles of Tai Chi and the special characteristics of each one.

Chen Lineage

Chen forms are done with changes of pace, stamping and dynamic tension, and there are sudden, sharp Fa Jin/Discharging Skilled Force movements. There is much twisting and vibrating to create Reeling Silk Skilled Force.

Of the variations on Chen style, the best known is the Tai Chi of Zhaobao, named after a town about 210km (130 miles) from Chen village. Its movements tend to be softer and slower than in the original Chen style and its applications seem largely based around locking techniques.

Zhaobao practitioners claim that their Tai Chi came from Zhang Sanfeng on Wudang Mountain and not from the Chens. Most unlikely. The Tai Chi masters on Wudang, dressed like Taoist priests with their mobile phones and iPads, are a new phenomenon.

Generally, in terms of stance work and the use of body torque/coiling, Chen style is taught to a higher level than the styles of the other four famous families. This is partly because its forms are more vigorous and so it appeals to a younger set.

Yang Lineage

All agree (so it's a known known) that Yang Luchan learned Tai Chi in the Chen village, in Henan province.

The consensus is that he came from a peasant family from Hebei province, Guangping prefecture, Yongnian county. He helped his father in the fields and, as a teenager, held various temporary posts. At one time he did odd jobs at the Tai He Tang Chinese Pharmacy in Yongnian City, owned by Chen Dehu from the Chen village.

One day Yang reportedly witnessed one of the partners of the pharmacy defeat a group of aggressors using Tai Chi Chuan. Impressed, he asked Chen Dehu to teach him. Chen reputedly sent Yang to the Chen village (a distance of nearly 300km/200 miles) to learn from his own teacher, Chen Changxing. Another version of the story is that Yang and his friend, Li Bokui, went to the Chen village as indentured servants.

When I visited the Yang family mansion in Guangping in 1997, I discovered their family's illustrated history was along the same lines, save that they say that, after an initial long sojourn in the Chen village, Yang Luchan returned home to Guangping. There he began to teach Tai Chi and raise a family. His eldest son, Yang Fenghou, was born in 1835, when Yang Luchan would have been in his mid-thirties. The Yang family story is that Yang went back to the Chen village twice to see his Tai Chi family and to improve his skills. Four of the five Tai Chi families acknowledge that Yang transmitted the art directly to them.

The Yang family and other Yang lineage systems teach a standardized Long Form, as well as Spear, Sabre and Sword Forms, the standard weapons in Chinese martial arts in general and Tai Chi in particular – see page 108. There are single- and double-hand Pushing Hands techniques as well as Da Lu/Big Sideways Diversion. Movements in Yang style tend to be large and expansive, so it is termed Big Frame Tai Chi. Generally the Hand Form is done slowly and softly, but some Yang schools occasionally do Fa Jin/Discharging Skilled Force movements when practising form.

So-called Classical Yang style is the final form of Yang Chengfu from the third generation of the Yang family. Yang Chengfu is credited with standardizing and popularizing most of the Yang style Tai Chi practised today. What few people are aware of is that Chinese martial arts historians are of the opinion that in the first three generations of Yang family there are at least four different Long Form variations of Yang style. Tai Chi continues to be passed down through the Yang family to the present day.

The Different Long Forms

In the syllabus of the Chen school today there are two Long Forms, the Tai Chi Form and the Pao Chui Form. We know that they are not the same as the two Long Forms which the Chens say Chen Changxing taught nearly 200 years ago.

We know this because it is well documented that the forms now practised in the village were revised by Chen Fake (1887–1957), who moved to Beijing and became the most famous Chen family master; by his top student, Feng Zhiqiang (1928–2012); and by the Chens themselves. The two forms can be Old Frame or New Frame or Small Frame or Big Frame, depending on the line of transmission. There are also applications for the techniques, but these are not taught at first.

There are five types of Pushing Hands in Chen style although, according to Feng Zhiqiang, in Chen Style Taijiquan these do not follow The 13 Tactics of Tai Chi Chuan, nor do they follow a fixed pattern.

Chen weapons include Single Sabre, Double Sabre, Single Sword, Double Sword, Double Mace, Pear Blossom Spear, White Ape Staff, Spring and Summer Halberd (in different weights) and Sticking Spears training.

The Long Forms practised by Yang lineage styles are fairly uniform in terms of names of the techniques, sequences and method of performance. Let us now compare these forms with those practised in the Chen family village.

The Yang lineage techniques Single Whip, Cloud Hands, Pat the Horse High and Fair Lady Works the Shuttle all occur in both the Chen Tai Chi Chuan and Pao Chui forms. The Chen form also includes White Crane Spreads Its Wings, Twist Step, Fist under Elbow, Fan through the Back, Wild Horse Parting Mane, Golden Cockerel on One Leg, Lotus Leg, Punch the Groin, Ride the Tiger and Tai Chi In Unity. The Pao Chui form includes Deflect, Parry and Forearm (instead of Deflect, Parry and Punch), and White Snake Puts Out its Tongue. There are also a few other techniques where there are similarities in the names between the various forms. For greater clarity, lists of these have been included in Appendix I (see page 233–5).

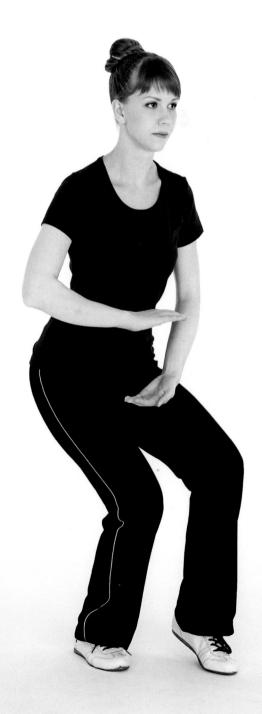

Right Pat the Horse High.

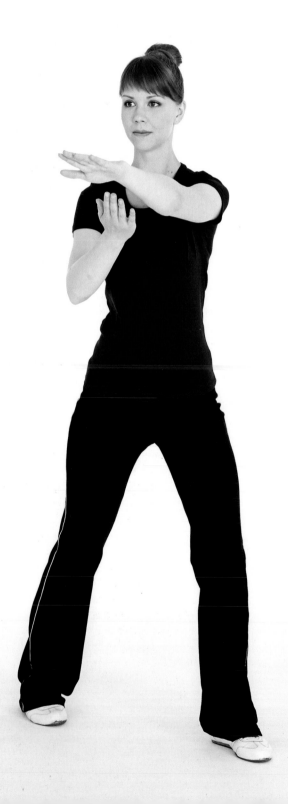

Yang techniques not found in Chen forms

Having identified certain similarities in the names of techniques, let us now look at differences. Yang lineage techniques such as Flying Oblique, Raise Hands Step Up, Stroking the Lute, Separating the Legs, Box the Ears, Snake Creeps Down and Slap the Face and inner form techniques, among others, are not found in the Chen forms. Again, a full list can be found in Appendix I (see pages 233–5).

The following Chen Tai Chi Form techniques do not occur in the Yang lineage forms: Buddha's Warrior Attendant Pounding Mortar, First Conclusion, Hidden Hand Punch, Bend Back and Use Shoulder, Blue Dragon Flies Up from the Water, Three Palm Changes, Retreat and Press Elbow, Rub the Foot, Hit Ground with Fist, Animal Head Posture, Hurricane Kick, Small Grasp and Hit, Double Snake Foot, White Ape Offers Fruit, Sparrow Ground Dragon and Face Opponent Cannon.

In the Chen Pao Chui Form, techniques which do not appear in the Yang lineage include Buddha's Warrior Attendant Pounding Mortar, Guard The Heart Punch, Attack Waist Press Elbow Punch, Wind Blowing Plum Blossoms, Hidden Body Punch, Turning Flowers Dancing Sleeves, Hidden Hand Punch, Continuous Cannon, Retreat Riding Unicorn, Firecracker on the Left and Right, Animal Head Posture, Fist Colours Eyebrow Red, Yellow Dragon Leaves Water, Sweep Ground With Leg, Rush On Left and Right, Four Hand Cannon and many others.

My conclusions are:

• That the Chens, through Chen Wangting, revised their Shaolin-influenced Pao Chui to include almost all of the names and in some cases also the applications of *The Classic of Boxing* techniques.

• About 200 years later, Tai Chi came to the village from an outsider, probably Jiang Fa, who taught Chen Changxing. Chen mixed in some of the best Chen Hand Form techniques (including some with the same names as techniques in *The Classic of Boxing*) with the new Tai Chi Long Form, creating a hybrid, at least as far as Hand Form was concerned. This is what Yang Luchan learned and took away with him to Guangping and Beijing.

• The Chens continued to practise Pao Chui, but they reinforced it with the new Tai Chi moves.

I have to confess that this is not the conclusion I was looking for. I wanted a 'pure', 'Taoist' art of Tai Chi. But the evidence is overwhelming. I can only agree with Sherlock Holmes's dictum that, once you have eliminated the impossible, whatever is left, however improbable, must nevertheless be the truth.

It's a bit of a mess and none of the famous Tai Chi families comes out of it with honour.

Going beyond Hand Forms, my Sifu's version of the Yang lineage syllabus has eight major methods of Pushing Hands and many variations; there are 24 Yin and Yang Neigong exercises, and 48 major San Shou fighting techniques, including Five Element Arm, Running Thunder Hand and Flying Flower Palm, which are not named in any Hand Form. The Sword, Sabre and Spear Forms and techniques are radically different from those of the Chen style. Finally, the Yang lineage Tai Chi systems have many other concepts and writings to which the Chens do not subscribe.

Yang Practice in Private

The way the Yangs practise in private is very different to the standardized way they teach at seminars. I'm grateful to my old Teutonic chum, Cordyline Batz, for this information. I first met him in Yongnian in 1997 at the annual Tai Chi festival, when I managed to irritate the chief organizer by chewing gum and performing Tai Chi at the same time. Cordy spent many months there, training with the Yang family.

They practise Long Form three times consecutively wearing lead-weighted suits, completing the form in around ten minutes each time.

They also practise a Pao Chui/Cannon Punch form that is different from the Chen Pao Chui. I talked with All China Champion Wang Haijun about this many years back and we agreed that this was probably a recent development.

They also practise a Wu Yuxiang form – this is extraordinary, as Wu was a student of the first two generations of Yang family. Contrary to all Chinese views on hierarchy, we have the masters learning from their students, though in terms of social class, the Wus were gentry and the Yangs were peasants – another paradox.

The Yangs practise their Hand Form with jump kicks; some techniques have multiple variations.

Yang Offshoots

There are a number of popular offshoots of Yang Style. The best known is Cheng Man-ching style, which is understated, Small Frame and very erect. Cheng (1902–75) became very successful, partly because of his connections with the Nationalist (Guomindang) party – the ruling party of Taiwan, where he moved in 1949 – but more because of Robert W Smith's writings, which greatly boosted Cheng's reputation in the West. He relocated to America in 1964, where he became an overnight success.

Robert W Smith was a CIA desk jockey who took up Chinese martial arts when he was posted to Taiwan in 1959; specifically he trained in Tai Chi with Cheng Man-ching, who'd been a student of Yang Chengfu for about six years. (When I visited the Yang family museum, however, Cheng was not listed as one of Yang Chengfu's disciples.) It's known that Cheng trained for some time with Zhang Qinlin and a mysterious Taoist; he also practised a secret Qigong. He was very reticent about these matters.

Cheng was not just an ordinary Guomindang member, he also taught painting to Soong Mei-ling, wife of the Guomindang leader Chiang Kai-shek, and was one of Chiang's personal physicians. Given their respective backgrounds, it's not surprising that Cheng and Smith became a team.

My Sifu remembered meeting Cheng Man-ching in Taiwan in 1957: they pushed hands for some minutes. His impression was that Cheng was very soft, but not very martial. Cheng did, however, give Sifu one of his paintings.

Another Yang offshoot is the Tung/Dong style, from Dong Yingjie (1898–1961), who practised first Hao style, then Yang style. He was famous for his fast Hand Form and the splayed hand/open palm position.

Next is Yang Jia Michuan/Yang Family Secret Transmission, from Wang Yennian (1914–2008), who learned from Zhang Qinlin. Zhang won the Chinese national fighting championship and was said to have been rewarded by being taught a special Yang family Hand Form and Sword Form, for successfully accepting a challenge on his teacher's behalf. One of this style's characteristics is that the weight is kept on the back foot most of the time.

I interviewed Wang in France back in 1999, having been introduced by an old chum, Claudy Jeanmougin. Wang well remembered Cheng Man-ching and 'Smifu' (Wang's rendition of 'Smith'). He told me that the reason Cheng's students didn't reach his level was that he didn't teach: when there were Pushing Hands challengers, Cheng would send for Wang.

It was Yang Jianhou, his son Yang Chengfu, and their committed students who did most to popularize Tai Chi – but as an art good for health.

Wu Lineages

Wu Jianquan

The Wus are the only famous Tai Chi family who are not ethnic Chinese. They adopted the Chinese family name of Wu, which sounded similar to their original Manchurian name. The first of the family to learn Tai Chi was Wu Quanyou (1834–1902), a senior student of Yang Luchan. He and his son Wu Jianquan (1870–1942) were hereditary Manchu cavalry officers of the Yellow Banner and the Imperial Guard.

At the time many Manchu princes in the Forbidden City studied martial arts, in particular Tai Chi Chuan, in order to improve their health. They were taught by Yang Luchan and his son, Yang Banhou. Because only Manchu princes or guards of the royal household learned Tai Chi, everyone thought that it was an aristocratic art. Tai Chi was developed and practised by the Yang and Wu families inside the Forbidden City for almost half a century.

Towards the end of his life, Wu Quanyou moved his family back to his ancestral home in Da-xing district in Hebei. He taught his son, Wu Jianquan, in a severe way. Wu Jianquan was originally employed by the Qing court in a palace battalion of the Imperial Guards. After Emperor Puyi abdicated in 1912, Chief of General Staff Yin Chang recommended Wu Jianquan to President Li Yuan Hong. In 1914, Wu was appointed to the 11th Corps of the Presidential Bodyguard as military instructor and martial arts advisor. Among his students were many of the Chiefs of Staff.

Wu Jianquan modified the forms he had studied and invented Square Form as an introduction to the Round Form. There are claims that he removed jumps and broken rhythm from the Hand Form, though such moves were kept in weapon forms and in Pushing Hands. Some claim that he used a narrower circle and created many new ways to apply the forms in a practical manner. In 1916, Wu Jianquan, along with Yang Shaohou, Yang Chengfu, Sun Lutang and Xu Sheng, founded a martial arts school in Beijing. Tai Chi Chuan, once reserved for royalty and military men, was now made available to the general public. So Tai Chi came to be taught by warriors for health.

The Institute recruited more than 60 students from the teaching ranks of high schools and universities throughout Beijing. Wu family third-generation brothers Wu Kungyi and Wu Kungcho were among the first graduates. The Institute's excellent results won praise from the Beijing University Dean, who recommended to the Ministry of Education that it be moved to a new location and expanded. So the Beijing Institute of Physical Education was born. Students were selected from the provinces to train at the school for two years before returning home to become martial arts teachers. This helped to spread Wu-style Tai Chi throughout China. Wu Jianquan was also asked to teach Tai Chi at the famous Jing Wu martial arts school in Shanghai.

Wu Jianquan is said to have trained in 1909 with the enigmatic Song Shuming, who had been Secretary to General Yuan Shikai, self-proclaimed emperor for three months in 1915–16. Song Shuming's influence could explain differences in the Wu school syllabus compared with the Yang.

Northern Wu Style

The so-called Northern/Beijing Wu style was passed down to Wang Peisheng, who wasn't considered much of a fighter. Rather, he focused on micro-teaching of Tai Chi with reference to acupoints among other things. Wang's books and videos feature unrealistic applications, but he had good posture.

Wu's daughter, Yinghua, and her husband, Ma Yueliang, took over in Shanghai. Yinghua was orthodox with fine posture, but her technique was lacking in body torque. Ma was into empty force and taught a fast form that he said was part of the Wu lineage. Nobody outside of Ma's school really believes this, though it's a nice form.

Hong Kong Wu Style

There are three versions of Hong Kong Wu style. The first is from Wu Kungyi and is very Small Frame. Stances are high and kicks are low. It isn't impressive. However, Wu Kungyi was the last master from the famous families to be involved in a punch-up; when in his mid-fifties he fought the much younger Chan Hak-fu of White Crane Boxing in a public challenge match. He made Chan's nose bleed. The fight was abandoned.

The second version is similar to the first and came from my Sifu's uncle, Cheng Wing-kwong. It is neat but understated.

The final version of Hong Kong Wu style is from my Sifu's main tutor, Qi Minxuan, whose father trained with Wu Quanyou. It's Medium to Large Frame, with a strong martial emphasis. Unusually for a Yang lineage method, the forms are done with changes of pace. *The Tai Chi Chuan Discourse* compares Tai Chi to the great river, the Changjiang. The speed of a river's flow changes in accordance with the terrain it passes through. In Tai Chi practice the speed of a form should change in accordance with the nature of the techniques being performed. Qi Minxuan was a great believer in the use of body and limb torque.

Many students from this school became international full-contact champions and I still occasionally get students who want to take this path, as I did myself.

Hong Kong Wu schools all teach Square Form to beginners. This is basic movement, like block letters, and acts as an introduction to the more sophisticated Round Form. Hong Kong Wu seems to be alone in practising the 24-exercise Neigong.

This Wu lineage is second only to the Yang in popularity. It is more extreme in terms of weight distribution – 10 per cent empty foot, 90 per cent substantial foot – but essentially the Long Form is the same as that of the Yangs.

Some of the worst Tai Chi can be found in the Wu lineage (I don't exempt my own school from this criticism); partly because of the influence of Square Form, exponents fail to use body torque and there isn't enough contrast between closing and opening techniques.

My Sifu once had an altercation with Wu Kungyi while pushing hands. He footswept Wu to the ground; Wu swore at my Sifu, who told Wu that his Kung Fu was in his mouth, not his hands. He never went back and never used the name Wu style after that, though his uncle was loyal to the Wu family to the end.

The Other Wu Lineage

Before Yang Luchan arrived in Beijing in 1852, he met and taught Tai Chi to the three Wu brothers in Yongnian. This Wu family is often confused with the Wu lineage mentioned earlier, but the characters for their names are both very dfferent. We don't know how much the Wu brothers learned or for how long they were with Yang. We do know that they were somehow involved in the discovery of The Tai Chi Chuan Classics and perhaps even wrote some of them.

The Wu Yuxiang style has high stances and neat upright postures with limited body torque. Movements are not expansive. The standard Long Form follows the same sequence as the regular Yang with a few differences such as jump kicks and the technique Green Dragon Coming Out of the Water, which don't exist in the Yang Long Form.

The lineage went through the Wu brothers to their nephew, Li Yiyu, and from him to Hao Weizhen (1842–1920), so this lineage is sometimes called Hao style. One of Hao's students was Sun Lutang (1860–1933).

Sun Style

Sun Lutang was a writer and scholar, already skilled in Baguazhang/Eight Trigram Boxing and Xingyi/Form and Intent Boxing, before he started training in Tai Chi under Hao Weizhen when he was in his early fifties. He made it his own by blending in elements of Baguazhang and Xingyi. He is credited with being the first to identify Tai Chi, Bagua and Xingyi as sister arts and to classify them as Nei Jia Chuan/Internal Family Boxing and Wudang, as opposed to External Boxing and Shaolin. This division is somewhat inaccurate, but rather useful, as in their theory and practice these arts do have similarities.

Sun was subsequently invited by Yang Shaohou, Yang Chengfu and Wu Jianquan to join them on the faculty of the Beijing Institute of Physical Education, where they taught Tai Chi to all comers. Sun taught there until 1928. This shows that the heads of three of the five Tai Chi families were on good terms and one wonders to what extent they influenced one another's approach.

My friend Bob Melia, long-time Chen and Sun stylist, believes that you need a foundation in Bagua and Xingyi to get the Sun-style structure right and to have penetration with techniques. Unfortunately these qualities are lacking in many Tai Chi practitioners, regardless of style. Sun's writings made his Tai Chi popular and it still retains the neat and compact look of Wu Yuxiang/Hao style.

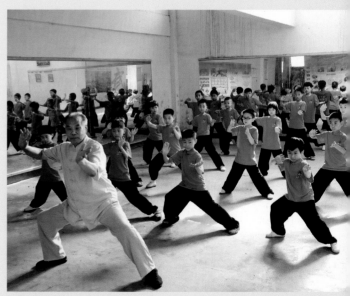

Above Chen-style class.

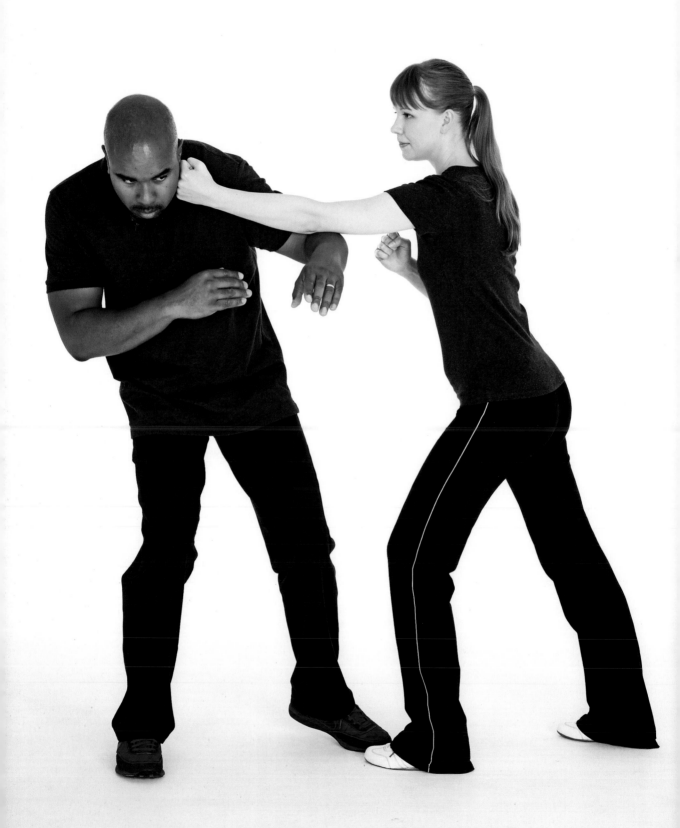

4 The Lost Drills of Tai Chi

In any kind of physical activity, and that includes Tai Chi, repetition of what the Chinese call Jibengong/Basic Skills is essential. The practical Tai Chi drills I'm introducing to you here are unknown unknowns for most people, even in my Sifu's own lineage. For most of the few dozen people who've learned them, they are unknown knowns: people don't understand either the drills or their many nuances. They come from my Sifu's second Sifu, the laconic Qi Minxuan. They're highly effective and great fun to practise.

Technique deteriorates under pressure, so the more gung-ho student may want to try out these drills against an opponent in a more spontaneous format such as free Pushing Hands training or full-contact sparring.

Running Thunder Hand

The name gives the clue. This is a dynamic, versatile striking drill which you can do with your palms or your fists; palms may be preferable if you are aiming to strike the large bones in the face. Begin with the left foot forward, facing your partner in a short front stance – though you may prefer your partner to face away from you, as it is less confrontational.

We'll start with a five direct strike pattern, as in Western Boxing, leading with the front hand, in this case the left (the reason I'm telling you to start with the front hand is reach – it's nearer to the opponent). Step in when you hit: to give the technique momentum, you need to move the feet.

The first strike is to the opponent's left eye, then to his nose, right eye, left jaw and right jaw. When you feel like it, change feet. This time, the lead hand will be the right, so the first strike is to the opponent's right eye, then to his nose, left eye, right jaw and left jaw. If you're using the fist rather than the palm, you can make the punch more effective by twisting the arm on impact, however this is a cruel and violent technique only to be used in extreme circumstances. When I was badly hurt in the Fourth Southeast Asian Chinese Pugilistic Championships in Singapore in 1976, I used this tactic to slice open cuts above and below both my Shaolin opponent's eyes. The referee stopped the fight.

Direct strike patterns

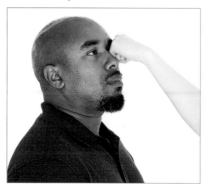

1. Strike left eye with left hand.

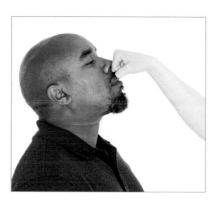

2. Strike nose with right hand.

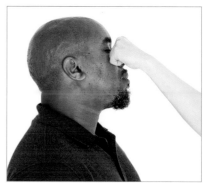

3. Strike right eye with left hand.

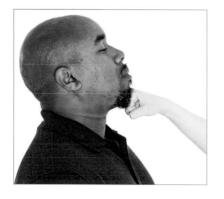

4. Strike left jaw with right hand.

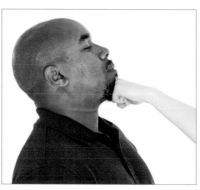

5. Strike right jaw with left hand.

Top tip

- The strength comes from the spine, so incline your weight forward to make your strikes stronger. Rotate the centre line (and therefore the spine) each time you strike.

Slicing strike patterns

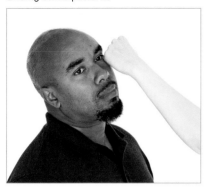

1. Strike left eye with left hand.

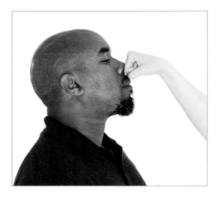

2. Strike nose with right hand.

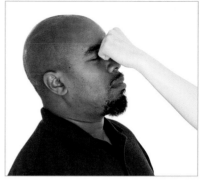

3. Strike right eye with left hand.

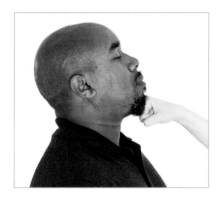

4. Strike left jaw with right hand.

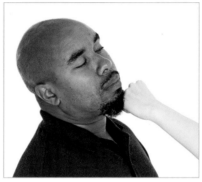

5. Strike right jaw with left hand.

Top tips

- There are hard bones in the head which can damage your hands if the impact is incorrect; if you feel unsure, use the palm rather than the fist when hitting your opponent's face.

- Lean the body weight forward into the punches; this will make them much stronger.

Now we are going to do circular slicing punches with the same five-strike pattern, leading with the front hand, in this case the left. The punches are anti-clockwise. Punches one, three and five slice across the target points from inside to out; punches two and four, with the right hand, are more direct. The striking sequence is the same as when we had the left foot forward with the direct strikes. The striking hand always comes over the other arm when that arm is retracted.

Change feet. Now we lead with the right hand and the punches go clockwise. Punches one, three and five are slicing across the target points from inside to out; punches two and four, with the left hand, are more direct. The striking sequence is the same as when we had the right foot forward with the direct strikes.

We can also practise Running Thunder Hand while holding light weights – I use 1.8kg (4lb) ones. Do 150 punches a minute for between 5 and 20 minutes. This will make your punches and palm strikes faster and more penetrating. This is what *An Interpretation of the Practice of the 13 Tactics* refers to as Fa Jin/ Discharging Skilled Force. It will also strengthen your grip.

When I did Chinese full-contact fighting at a competitive level, we'd start training about a hundred days before the competition. Each day I'd do 3,000 Running Thunder Hand punches with a 1.8kg (4lb) weight in either hand. I'd also do around a thousand punches on the heavy bag and the same on a focus mitt. Come the competition, I had half a million Running Thunder Hands in the bank. People wonder why there have been so few successful Tai Chi fighters. It's very simple: they're either doing the wrong kind of training or the right kind of training, but not enough of it, or they are temperamentally unsuited to this kind of activity. If you go to YouTube you can watch me do a Running Thunder Hand on big Roy Pink of Five Ancestors Kung Fu back in 1980.

We can also practise Running Thunder Hand as a reverse punch or cross, as it is called in boxing. This means if the left foot is forward, your cross will be with your right hand and vice versa.

This time your partner is going to run backward in a circle, holding up the hand (with or without focus pad) that's on the outside of the circle. You stride after him, punching with the reverse hand with each stride. You should be inclined forward so that when you step and transfer the weight your total body force is going into each strike; for added power, turn your body as you hit. The arms also make a partial rotation on impact, making each strike more penetrating. This is what *The Canon of Tai Chi Chuan* is getting at when it refers to Zou/Moving – we don't stand still when we're using Jin.

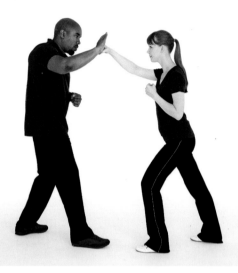 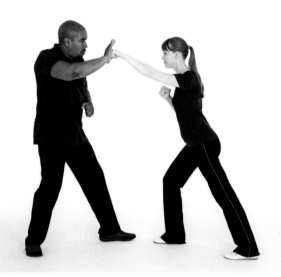

1. Step forward with the left foot and hit with the right hand.

2. Step forward with the right foot and hit with the left hand.

Putting It into Practice

Let's use Running Thunder Hand now in practical application. Both we and the opponent have got our guards up and left foot forward. We suddenly close the gap between us by stepping in with the front foot – in this case the left (in boxing this is called the drop step). Simultaneously we use a slicing Running Thunder Hand with our lead left hand, aimed at the opponent's head. If he doesn't block, he'll be hit. He blocks. As we retract the lead hand, we drag his block away and hit him with a Running Thunder Hand cross with our reverse hand. This is the killer punch.

Change the front foot. You are going to do the same thing again, coming now to the inside of the opponent's guard from time to time and getting him to do the same. The technique works equally well whether you're on the inside or the outside of the opponent's guard.

Top tips

• Keep the non-punching hand ready for action tucked under the chin.

• When retracting the non-striking hand, bring it directly under the chin so it is in the most advantageous place for follow-up action.

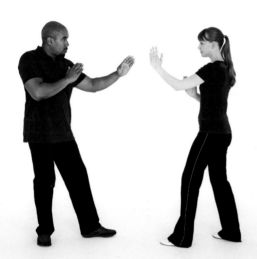

1. Face your opponent in a Seven Star guard (see page 176) just out of striking range.

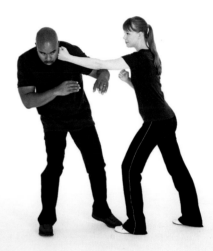

2. Step in with the front foot, using the drop step, and slice across to your opponent's head with the front hand.

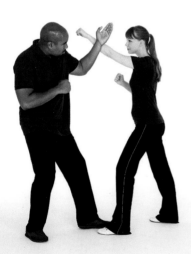

3a. Your opponent blocks the strike.

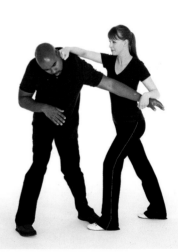

3b. Retract your punching arm, keeping contact with his blocking arm and pulling that back too, opening him up for a cross/reverse punch with your other fist.

Flying Flower Palm

The character for flower sounds similar to Hua, meaning to transform, which is what we are trying to do here, so translating it as 'flower' may be an error. This little-known drill is all about duality. We practise four pairs of open-hand strikes against a target such as a tree or hand or punch ball. This can be done one-handed or double-handed and the strikes can be defensive or offensive.

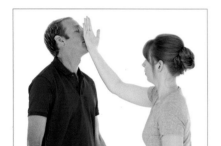

1. First duality – Yin palm.

2. First duality – Yang back of hand.

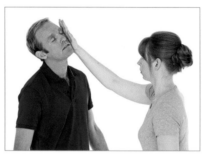

3. Second duality – forehand coming across.

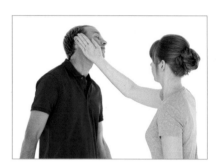

4. Second duality – backhand slaps across.

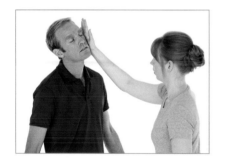

5. Third duality – slap on his left.

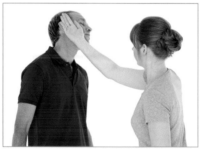

6. Third duality – slap on his right.

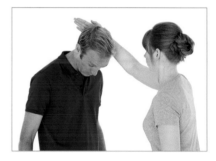

7. Fourth duality – closing palm.

Let's start by using one hand. If the left foot is forward, we'll use the lead left hand. The first duality is Yin/Yang. The palm is soft, so it's Yin. The back of the hand is hard, so it's Yang. The movement is forward-directed: a palm strike followed by a strike with the back of the hand.

The second duality is Jing Fan. Jing is orthodox, while Fan is reverse. It's a bit like forehand and backhand in tennis. Jing is a palm strike, while Fan is a strike with the back of the hand.

The third duality is simply Left and Right. It doesn't really matter which hand we begin with and we can use either the palm or the back of the hand for each strike.

The fourth and final duality is He Kai, Close and Open. Closing involves slapping the opponent round the back of the head; this means your palm strike is coming towards you. Opening therefore involves a forward-directed palm strike or slap with the back of the hand.

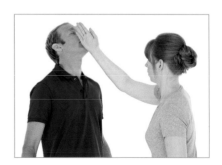

8. Fourth duality – opening palm.

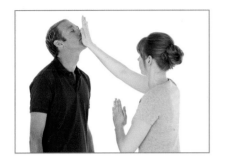

1. First duality – Yin right palm.

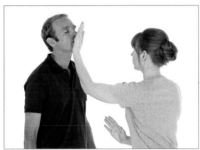

2. First duality – Yang left palm.

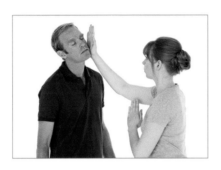

3. Second duality – right forehand coming across.

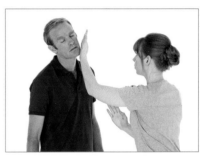

4. Second duality – left backhand slaps across.

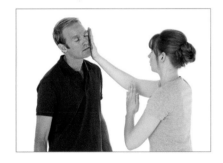

5. Third duality – right-hand slap on opponent's left.

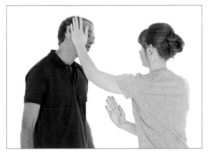

6. Third duality – left-hand slap on his right.

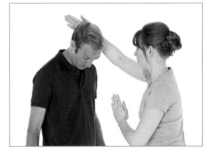

7. Fourth duality – closing right palm.

Once we are fluent on both the left and the right in using only one hand for the drill, we switch to using two hands alternately. We gradually build up speed as our fluency increases. The fundamental purpose of Flying Flower Palm is to train us in recovery and continuity. If we miss with one hand/one technique, we come back with another. This applies to striking techniques, grappling techniques and weapon techniques or to combinations thereof.

This skill is also linked to Reeling Silk, Pushing Hands and the concept of Gyrating Arms.

Last week I was up in Edinburgh working with my old pal Jimmy Connachan and his students, including Nan and her chums (see page 87), none of whom will see 70 again. They had big fun doing Flying Flower Palm on me.

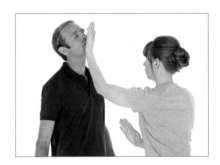

8. Fourth duality – opening left back hand.

Five Element Arm

I first learned this drill in 1976 for a TV Tai Chi demo which was a backdrop to the 1976 Miss Universe contest in Hong Kong. My old training partner, Tong Chi-kin, and I began with this, then went through a host of Tai Chi throwing techniques to the sound of the Carl Douglas pop song 'Kung Fu Fighting'.

Despite the name, there is no tortuous logic tenuously linking Five Element Arm to Chinese philosophy's Five Element theory, except that in *The Tai Chi Chuan Discourse* the Five Elements are linked to stepping forward, back, left and right and having central equilibrium at all times when we apply the technique.

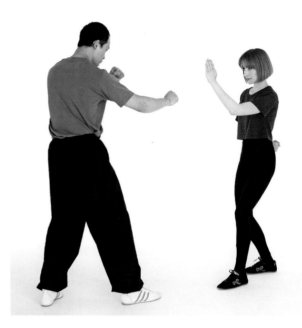

1. We'll begin with the left foot forward, which means we'll also start off using the left arm, as it's nearer to the opponent and we don't want to defend across the body. Note that the premise here is that the other arm is injured,the hand is in a pocket or the other arm is being held or is holding something (exactly my situation when I was attacked near my home many years ago).

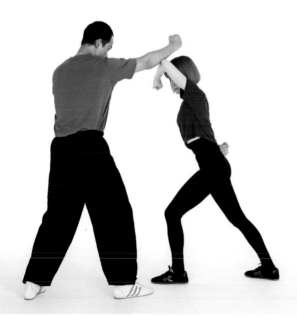

4. Next he tries an overhead hammer/axe strike down on the skull. We shift forward into it, lifting the left arm with the point of the elbow angled up. The harder he hits, the more the point of our elbow will hurt his arm on impact. At worst his arm will slide down the outside of our arm. We immediately counter with the left arm or with a kick.

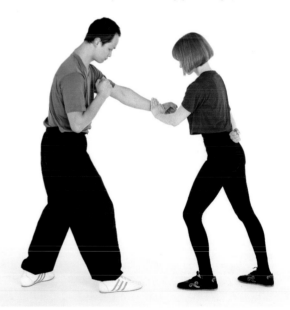

5. His next swing is to the left side of the body. We shift the feet, turn the body and bring the left arm down and across in a sliding impact. We then counter as before.

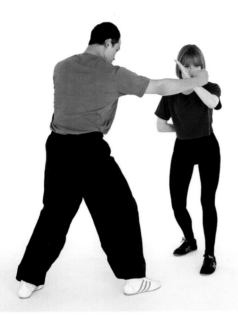

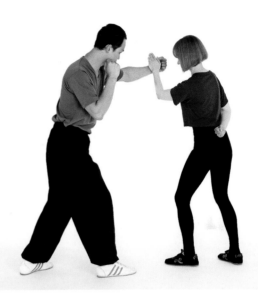

2. The opponent swings to the left side of the head; we turn and raise the left arm to give a sliding impact defence and counter him immediately with the left hand or a kick with either leg.

3. Now he swings to the other side of the head. We shift the feet and weight and turn, raising the left arm again to make a sliding impact and immediately counter as before.

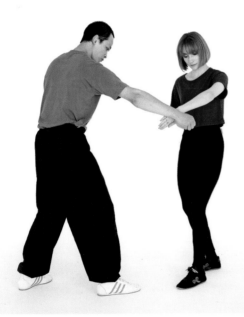

6. The final attack is to the right side of the body. We shift the feet, turn the body and use our left palm to make a brushing impact along his left arm to dissipate the force. We counter with the left hand or either foot at whatever target is most opportune; we must always be ready to follow up with another hit if required.

When you are clear about how to do the five defences your opponent will start attacking randomly, sometimes high, sometimes low. Never let him swing more than twice before making a counter. Once you are competent with the left arm, switch to using the right as before.

Top tip

• Each time you defend, move the feet to change the angle relative to your opponent, and to help absorb attacks.

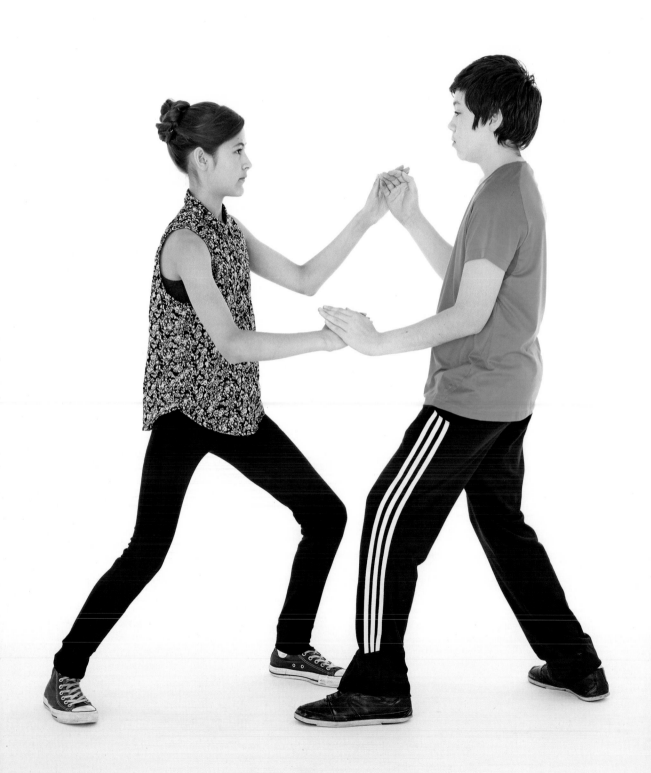

5 Physiology and the Benefits of Tai Chi

It's often said that practising Tai Chi is good for health, but it's all a bit vague. Here we'll look at the benefits more analytically.

Physiology

For many years, Tai Chi has been learned and taught with a strong emphasis on the notion that regular practice leads to improvements in one's health and warding off disease (in the Far East regular means daily; in the West it probably means once or twice a week). In Hong Kong, back in 1976, I went with my Sifu to meetings with the Sport and Recreation Department to discuss setting up Tai Chi classes in all the public housing estates in Hong Kong: the idea was to promote community well-being and reduce health costs. Many students from these classes went on to attend Tai Chi instructor courses, at the end of which their competence to teach basic Tai Chi for health would be tested. If successful they'd become certificated instructors. The project has been extremely popular.

The perceived health benefits of Tai Chi have often been explained with Traditional Chinese Medical concepts such as meridian theory, as used in acupuncture. There is also much reference to more abstract concepts such as Qi, Jing and Shen when dealing with aspects of internal alchemy. However, in the last few decades much of the anecdotal and subjective health benefits of Tai Chi has been investigated with scientific rigour. This is better than relying on the observations of the old masters, though it does not invalidate those masters' years of experience.

There are many different styles of and approaches to Tai Chi practice. It is likely that practising all the different individual aspects within one style or the same individual aspect in any style would have different effects on the student's health; then there are other variables such as duration and regularity of practice.

The Three Treasures of Chinese Internal Alchemy

In Wai Dan/Chinese external alchemy, drugs and herbs are used to produce an elixir; in Nei Dan/internal alchemy, the body uses Qi/Vital Energy (in the sense of breath and circulation), combined with Jing/Vital Essence (in the sense of bodily secretions) to produce an elixir internally, thereby purifying the Shen/Spirit. Qi, Jing and Shen are therefore known as the Three Treasures.

I've translated Qi as Vital Energy here, but this term does not convey the concept of Qi in its entirety. The character itself (opposite, left) represents rice being cooked in a pot and giving off vapour: this gives us the concept of alchemical change so beloved of the Taoists. Qi is many different things. There is Qi all around us: the air is Qi; the oxygen that we extract from the air is also Qi. The oxygen transported by haemoglobin which is delivered from the lungs to the tissues of the body is Qi. The carbon dioxide, oxygen and methane gas discharged from the body are also examples of Qi.

The character Shen (opposite, middle) represents on the left the sky and the various heavenly bodies and on the right two hands extending a rope, so there is the concept of expansion. The combination has man reaching for the stars, so perhaps Spirit or Spiritual Essence is the best translation in the present context.

The third treasure, Jing, means the Essence; it refers to semen and to vaginal and other bodily secretions. Again, the character (opposite, right) on the left depicts the rice plant, while on the right the upper part means to give birth and the lower represents the colour of the plants. Without a good supply of Qi, Jing is lacking and Shen cannot be at ease. If Shen is not tranquil, the breathing is adversely affected, as is the ability to produce or retain Jing.

As for the two types of alchemy, the Wai Dan process is outward and material and is said to transform the adept into an earthly immortal, whereas Nei Dan is inward and spiritual and turns the adept into a celestial immortal. The latter can then fly to the abode of the Jade Emperor, which is said to be rather splendid. Both processes were practised in seclusion – this often meant in the mountains. If you want to get the flavour of this, I recommend a trip to the wonderful Wudang Mountain.

Qi and Shen are referred to many times in The Tai Chi Chuan Classics, but the term Jing occurs only three times and each time as part of the compound term Jingshen – Essence combined with Spirit. By extension this has the sense of vigour. In *An Interpretation of the Practice of the 13 Tactics* the message each time is to train vigorously:

*'The body and the intent are solely concentrated on the Jingshen,
Not on the Qi.
If on the Qi, there'll be stagnation.'*

Laozi asked the adepts, 'By concentrating your Qi, can you be as supple as a baby?'

They thought they could. The aim of internal alchemy was not to stop ageing, but to promote reversion, regeneration and return by using physiological alchemy to make the three 'primary endowments' of Qi, Jing and Shen as perfect and pure as they were at the beginning of life, the sex act often played a part in such practises.

In Taoism, this is called Fan Lao Huan Tong, meaning to return from old age to a baby's state of energy and purity through Taoist practice. This refers again to the concept of the Dantian/Cinnabar Fields that we saw earlier (see page 39). *The Canon of Tai Chi Chuan* tells us that 'the Qi sinks to the Dantian'. The lower Dantian, just below the navel, is the one of most relevance to Tai Chi, though there are some who practise abstruse breathing methods, involving all three Cinnabar Fields.

It was said, 'Following Nature leads to common life and death, going against it leads to immortality.' This is a Taoist paradox.

Internal alchemy changed; from about 415 CE there was a desexualization whereby the emphasis moved to respiration and diet.

There is another problem with internal alchemy. Many of the 'leading authorities' on the subject are academics like the late great Joseph Needham; while they seem to understand the theory, their writings make it plain that their sexual experience was woefully lacking. It's like someone who's never done partner work, but only form, attempting to defend himself. There are two ways to circulate Qi in internal alchemy. The first is to use the intention to direct it to a particular place; this visualizing of the Qi flow was called an inner vision. The second way is to let the Qi take its normal course. The approach of some Taoists to their respiratory exercise was highly regulated as to time, place and so on. Some also used acupoints in their training. Sometimes such training could result in aerophagia (habitual swallowing of air) and flatulence. One imagines that at times this proved to be socially awkward.

The Tai Chi Chuan Discourse instructs us that 'the Qi should be excited to activity'. Whatever we do must therefore be lively.

An Interpretation of the Practice of the 13 Tactics encourages us to 'use the Xin/heart mind to move the Qi, try to let it sink in an orderly manner. Then it can accumulate and enter the bones. Use the Qi to move the body; try to let it move without hindrance.'

If we concentrate our minds on the movements and doing them correctly with closing and opening, contracting and expanding, both the breathing and the movements will become continuous and orderly.

As both Laozi and Zhuangzi were poking fun at Taoist adepts more than 2,000 years ago, it is clear that Chinese internal alchemy dates back to remote antiquity.

Below The Three Treasures

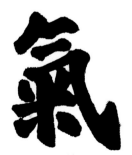

Qi – vital energy

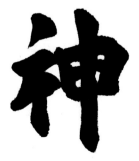

Shen – spiritual essence

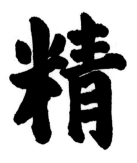

Jing – vital essence

Taoist Qigong

The Taoist approach to physiological alchemy included creating Golden Elixirs, sexual and respiratory techniques, massage, callisthenics and meditation. Meditation produced a tranquil mind, while diet and exercise healed the body. Most of these techniques can be found in one form or another in Tai Chi practice.

The earliest pictorial evidence we have of Qigong is on an untitled silk scroll found in one of the tombs at the archaeological site of Mawangdui in Hunan province. It dates from 168 BCE and depicts 28 exercises (originally there were 40, but 12 are now illegible). Both men and women, old and young, are shown exercising. The exercises include animal movements such as bird stretching and bear rambling as well as 'using the pole to contact Yin and Yang'. Some are of the exercises reminiscent of Tai Chi movements.

The physician Hua Tuo (c. 140–208 CE) and the philosopher Chen Tuan taught their own systems of Qigong. There were also many illustrated manuals on the subject.

The Chinese were obsessed with sex: done correctly, they maintained that it could extend your lifespan; done with frequent ejaculation, it shortened it. Also there was the problem of concubinage and trying to keep a number of different women satisfied (sexually at least). This meant that ejaculation control and stimulation techniques that could be acquired through Qigong practice became sought after skills.

When I learned Tai Chi Neigong, I was told not to ejaculate for a hundred days as the exercises would then be more effective. When I trained for full-contact competition, the rule was strictly no sex for at least three months. Finally, in the Taoist internal alchemy Qigong (not a Tai Chi method) that I practise, one exercise has the specific purpose of preventing ejaculation.

Peng Zu, a legendary long-lived culture hero, said to have lived more than 3,000 years ago, allegedly acquired his longevity by combining external and internal alchemy methods. Known as the Chinese Methuselah, he's said to have married more than a hundred wives and fathered hundreds of children, as late as in his 800s. Yes, eight hundreds. Hero indeed.

Peng Zu is said to have extended his lifespan by practising internal alchemy techniques to harvest and absorb the woman's energy during intercourse, while retaining his semen.

Is semen retention important?
Semen, we now know, contains prostaglandins, which have a powerful endocrine action, acting on an array of cells.

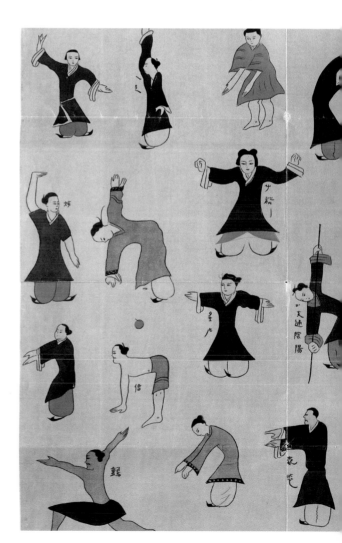

Right Exercise scroll from Mawangdui tomb.

They also:
- cause constriction of vascular smooth muscle cells
- cause aggregation and disaggregation of platelets
- sensitize spinal neurons to pain
- help to induce labour
- decrease intraocular pressure
- regulate inflammatory medication
- regulate calcium movement
- control hormone regulation
- control cell growth
- act on the hypothalamus to produce fever
- act on improving the function of cells in the kidneys
- act on parietal cells in the stomach wall to inhibit acid secretion.

It's clear that semen is a very potent substance. Many men fall asleep after ejaculation and there has to be a psychological consequence also. However, the general position of Western science is that it is not a problem for the body to generate more semen; it's just a matter of time.

There are essentially two approaches to semen retention. One is by internal alchemy exercises to prolong intercourse and prevent ejaculation. In this approach there is no male orgasm. The second is to block the seminal duct at the area of the perineum so that the semen is diverted into the bladder and is discharged on urination. I prefer the first method as I don't like the way the second approach overrides the autonomic nervous system; it is potentially dangerous and I've met a number of people who've had bad side effects from this practice. Adepts thought that the semen returned to nourish the brain; it seems they didn't know it went to the bladder. Some later made the excuse that by the time the semen went to the bladder, they had used its essence.

The Song of the 13 Tactics tells us, 'When the Wei Lu (coccyx acupoint) is centrally correct, the Shen connects with the headtop.' This is exactly the Taoist concept of nourishing the brain, although here the context is Tai Chi practice rather than sexual congress. It seems we need more detailed studies on the value of semen retention.

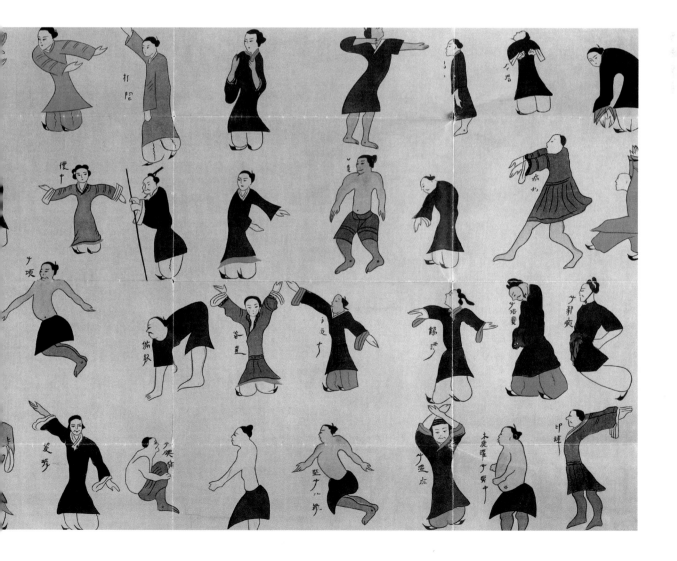

Health Benefits

Research has shown that regular Tai Chi practice confers many defined benefits to the various systems within the human body; the best book on the subject by far is the *Harvard Medical School Guide to Tai Chi*. Its research shows that body shape influences negotiations and changes the body's endocrine function and mood. It is clear that Tai Chi is a comprehensive method of exercise, which affects all of the body's systems, so let's examine each in turn.

Cardiovascular System

The movements of the Hand Form will naturally cause a gentle increase in the workload of the heart. Certain postures, such as raising the arms above the head, have additional effects such as stimulating the circulation. There are many different approaches to Tai Chi and the speed and depth at which forms are performed also can introduce an aerobic aspect to the conditioning of the cardiovascular system.

For these reasons, Tai Chi has been used in some heart rehabilitation programmes with good results.

There is evidence that regular Tai Chi practice lowers blood pressure, thus reducing the risk of heart conditions and stroke. Tai Chi also enhances exercise capacity in cases of cardiopulmonary disease, so it's good for rehabilitation following heart attacks and bypass surgery.

Respiratory System

Tai Chi practice places emphasis on the breath, particularly abdominal breathing. In most Tai Chi schools the breathing is in and out through the nose. The mucous membranes in the nose help to filter and warm the air before it enters the lungs. If you breathe in through the mouth, the air will be cold when it enters the lungs, making respiratory illnesses more likely. The vast majority of Tai Chi practitioners keep the mouth closed and exhale through the nose. However, Professor Douglas Wile's book *Tai Chi Touchstones: Yang Family Secret Transmissions* contains a text supposedly dictated by Yang Chengfu to one of his students; this has him saying that exhaling should be through the mouth. Whether Yang really said this or not, your guess is as good as mine.

The general method of practice encourages long, slow, deep breathing which improves the function of the diaphragm. Certain postures which elevate the arms also expand the upper lobes of the lungs. Tai Chi has been shown to increase the total capacity of the lungs and also the amount of air that can be inhaled or exhaled in a single breath.

The health of your breath could predict your lifespan, so Tai Chi's capacity to improve your breathing can possibly lengthen your life.

Research has also shown that Tai Chi practice improves the efficiency of the lungs in absorbing oxygen and expelling carbon dioxide. This has implications for people who smoke: the increased amount of air taken in due to the increase in lung capacity means smokers who practise Tai Chi will take more smoke into the lungs and be able to keep it there for longer. There are obvious health consequences.

Nevertheless, Tai Chi can help alleviate symptoms in respiratory diseases such as asthma and emphysema.

Gastrointestinal System

The combination of deep abdominal breathing and the contraction, expansion and twisting of the body during Tai Chi practice can have some profound effects on the internal organs.

The massaging effect and changes in intra-abdominal pressure help to stimulate blood supply to the internal organs, thus improving their efficiency. In addition to regulating bowel function, this has beneficial effects on the kidneys, liver, spleen and other glands that expedite absorption of nutrients and elimination of waste products.

Musculoskeletal System

The relaxed, expansive, contracting, twisting and sinking movements of Tai Chi provide a comprehensive total body exercise. As with any form of load-bearing exercise, it brings improvements in muscle development as well as loosening of the joints.

From the musculoskeletal point of view the constant changing of weight in Tai Chi strengthens the legs, the leg joints and the feet and makes them more flexible. Studies show that Tai Chi helps with torso flexibility, while good alignment and correct use of core muscles and the spine help to make you more erect. Tai Chi breathing also acts as an internal massage and reduces musculoskeletal pain.

Tai Chi also has more subtle benefits, especially for those who are older or who require a more rehabilitative approach. Research has shown increases in both bone and bone marrow density with longer term practice. The total body alignment and movement principles also combine with increases in proprioception (awareness of the relative position of different parts of the body) to enhance mobility. This can be extended to those who are at risk of falls, such as the elderly and those suffering from Parkinson's disease and other conditions which affect the balance.

Neurological System

Alignment of the spine and stretching of different combinations of muscles and joints often have a stimulating effect on the nervous system. The correct holding of certain postures can also have profound neurological effects. This is especially true of the autonomic nervous system which has many regulatory effects on all the body's systems.

The way in which Tai Chi is practised can also have a meditative aspect. These benefits, in addition to the physical benefits mentioned earlier, have been shown to help with anxiety and insomnia.

Specific Medical Conditions

Parkinson's Disease and Cerebral Palsy

There has been one study of reasonable rigour showing that Tai Chi practice has definite benefits to those with these conditions, due to increased muscle strength, joint mobility, proprioception and autonomic feedback on the neurological system. I have experience teaching students with cerebral palsy in Sweden and they greatly enjoyed Pushing Hands, though we had to sit down to do it.

With specific reference to Parkinson's disease, one study showed that twice-weekly Tai Chi classes were much better than strength-building exercises or stretching for improving balance and motor control. Tai Chi has also been shown to increase tactile acuity, so Pushing Hands training should be of particular help in this regard.

I was diagnosed with Parkinson's disease in 2011 and can testify that it was only my daily Tai Chi sessions of Neigong and Running Thunder Hand training with a 1.8kg (4 lb) weight in each hand that got me through two years without medication. I take medication now, but the daily Tai Chi sessions give me a better quality of life than I'd have by medication alone.

Please be clear, however: I always practised Tai Chi because I just loved doing it. Even now I do it for fun and because I've loved martial arts since I was a kid.

Asthma

The positive effects of Tai Chi practice on lung capacity will affect measurements of asthma such as tidal volume and peak expiratory flow. Tai Chi can't cure asthma, but it does improve basic respiratory capacity. The same goes for emphysema. I have taught many asthmatics and after a few weeks of Tai Chi practice many no longer need their inhalers. Indeed, Tai Chi breathing is believed to activate the parasympathetic nervous system, which deals with the body's activities when at rest and therefore helps to regulate breathing.

Arthritis

There is some good research on the benefits of Tai Chi on osteoarthritis (especially of the knee) – this has been strongly linked to multiple studies on falls in the elderly. Tai Chi practice is the number-one most effective method of fall prevention.

Osteoporosis

There are also good studies showing significant improvements in bone density resulting from Tai Chi practice, but it would be very difficult to show a difference between this and other load-bearing e xercises in isolation.

Bowel Complaints and Indigestion

Constipation is the obvious one here. There have been studies (though not of sufficient rigour to be entirely convincing) suggesting that Tai Chi has some effect on inflammatory and irritable bowel disease. However, this may be due to background improvements on the immune system -- and it's difficult to isolate this improvement from dietary factors.

Insomnia

The neurological and meditative aspects of Tai Chi training probably help in dealing with insomnia, but there's no good quality evidence regarding Tai Chi alone – this research is mixed in with Qigong, Yoga and other meditative work.

What we *can* say is that Tai Chi may reduce the effects of stress and anxiety and in the workplace has been shown to improve health and psychological well-being. Tai Chi, as the Chinese have always known, is part of a lifestyle package.

Ages and Stages

Perhaps the most profound changes that Tai Chi brings about come from the combined improvements to the person as a whole. For example, stimulation of the neurological, vascular and glandular organs has additional effects on the immune system. In this way, Tai Chi can certainly provide a balanced and cohesive system of improving one's health.

'Chang Sheng bu Lao' – Long Life not Old

Pregnancy

In Hong Kong my Sifu's second wife taught Tai Chi to many pregnant women, as I have done myself; I also taught my son's mother when she was expecting and many other pregnant ladies. Tai Chi practice during pregnancy is extremely beneficial to the expectant mother and her unborn child. It stimulates the immune system, the circulation and nervous system of both mother and baby. In addition, it flexes the mother's spine. In the very late stages, it is advisable to stick to holding static postures, slow practice and basic Pushing Hands drills. Sudden movements are to be avoided. It is perfectly safe to practise in this way all through pregnancy.

Seniors

Tai Chi changes lives. My ex-wife's mother, Mrs Wong, fled to Hong Kong from China and ended up living with her husband and six children in a tiny flat in the soulless So Uk housing estate in Kowloon. Then one day in 1976, she heard a Tai Chi class was starting up, sponsored by the Hong Kong Government Sport and Recreation Department. She went along. She learned the Long Form. She learned the Sabre Form. She learned and loved above all the Sword Form. As a tailor she spent much of her life bent over sewing. Suddenly her posture improved, her health got better. She started going to tea with her Tai Chi friends. Her Sifu was one of my Tai Chi brothers and she always used to ask me for tips. She became his top student and assistant. My daughter Ellen has inherited her grandmother's sword.

I taught Tai Chi for a few years at the world-famous Budokwai Judo Club in London. One night an old gentleman turned up, carrying a stick and wearing a jacket and tie. He'd come the previous week in my absence, but my friend and assistant Cliff had told him that it was quite a martial class and perhaps not suitable.

I took a shine to the old gent, who turned out to be 71 years old, with severe mobility problems and a thirst for vodka which he believed his much younger and somewhat shrewish wife couldn't smell on his breath. He was a great student. I guess he knew he was in the last-chance saloon, so he was motivated. I taught him to stand. I taught him to move. After six weeks he could climb the steps to the practice hall without a stick. He told me he was practising twice a day every day and had cut down on the wine, women and song. Especially the song.

Tai Chi has been shown to reduce pain and stiffness in cases of arthritis. It can be taught as an aerobic activity of low to moderate intensity. Evidence supports the idea that Tai Chi improves aerobic capacity and arrests its decline in healthy older adults – in other words, it helps keep you fit.

Even standing still doesn't really happen, because maintaining any upright posture requires continuous effort and structure. Muscles need to be activated to keep the skeleton upright and in position. At the same time we continue with our normal functions such as breathing, swallowing, blood and lymph flow and the passing of gas.

The major reason for seniors having to attend Accident and Emergency units in hospitals is injuries incurred in falls, especially bone injuries. This is why the US Surgeon General specifically recommends Tai Chi for fall prevention; it also helps to maintain bone mass density, so the bones are less brittle and less likely to be injured in a fall.

Tai Chi trains the coordination of neuromuscular systems and improves balance when on the move. Evidence shows that is also reduces fear of falling by increasing body awareness, while improving the sensory systems and hence the balance. Studies show that Tai Chi practitioners have better foot alignment than age-matched non-practitioners.

All my Tai Chi life, I've emphasized foot and stance work; I was not wrong.

It is an easy lie to say that seniors don't like martial Tai Chi; I know many who love it. They punch with torque; they spin and slice with their swords. They may have come to Tai Chi late in life, but they enjoy it and are big fun to teach.

My old Sifu found living in Hong Kong increasingly unpleasant while suffering from congenital diabetes, so in his mid-fifties he moved back to his village in China. Over the course of the next 20 years his condition gradually worsened. He became blind and he could hardly walk. When I went to see him a few years before his death, I noticed that there was a rope attached to the bars of a window and a leather belt attached to the rope. I asked him what it was for.

He told me that he deeply regretted not having kept up his practice in his later years. All he could really do by that stage was Neigong, but he needed to wear the belt attached to the rope as it was the only way he could keep his balance. In some conditions, including diabetes, there is reduced sensation in the feet. Studies have shown that Tai Chi practice increases the sensitivity of the soles and positively affects walking speed and balance. For my Sifu it was too late.

Children

For a couple of years, back in the early 1970s, I taught Karate to kids from the age of seven upwards. It was both rewarding and challenging. Trying to teach Tai Chi to kids is more challenging still. The younger ones generally find Tai Chi Hand Form training hard going; it isn't lively enough for them. When teaching children I always show them a lot of partnered drills and applications, but avoid techniques such as joint locks which can damage young bodies.

An hour-long class is generally enough for most kids, but teenagers can manage longer. For many years I trained up youngsters for competition. It was very rewarding and some of them achieved redemption from poor choices they had made in their lives.

I taught my daughter Ellen Tai Chi from the age of three, starting with handstands, spear, footwork and punching. She attended lots of classes and camps and competed a few times. Now she trains sport fencing.

My son Ronan, I sent to Judo when he was three years old. The Judo folk are great with kids and teach them to look after themselves and give them a bit of discipline. Ronan also did a few years of sports fencing and learned some nifty moves. Now he enjoys Tai Chi weapon and hand applications and Pushing Hands. He's been training with adults since he was ten. I taught karate to kids when I was 19 years old myself, and I learned how to ride a bicycle for the first time at the age of 50, so I have few illusions about the differing learning capacities of young and old. The earlier you start, the sooner you begin to develop muscle memory and technique.

Below Edinburgh Tai Chi chums; left to right Edith, Margaret and Nan.

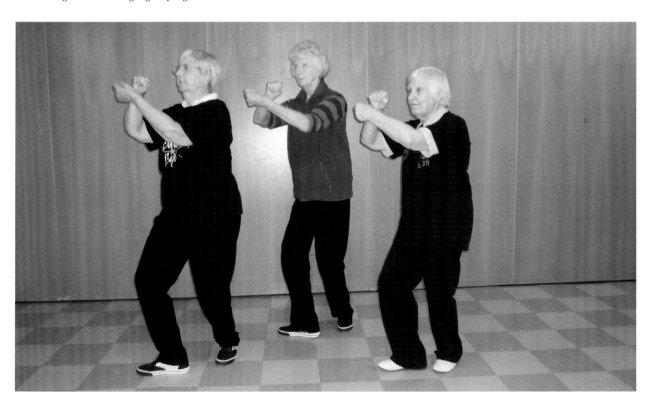

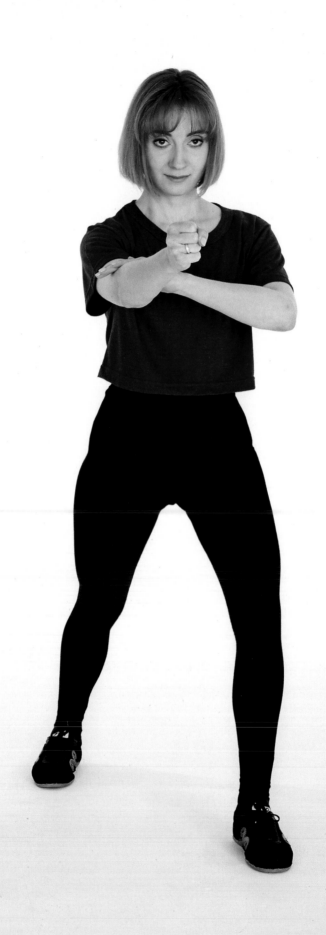

6 Fundamentals of Practice

In this section we'll discuss where we want to go with our Tai Chi and what fundamental things we'll need to do in each aspect of our practice in order to get there.

From the beginning, correctness of posture and stance is vital if you are to be able to move in a balanced and coordinated way. You need to learn to use the centre line (that is, the spine) to rotate and/or flex when you move. If you want to learn distance and timing, you'll need to do partner work such as Pushing Hands and application training.

Training Journeys

Former British international Karate competitor Terry O'Neill once said that he'd tried and enjoyed Tai Chi, but he felt that, unlike Karate, it was something that you had to practise every day and he just didn't have the time. Terry was probably right: daily practice is essential if you are to reach and maintain a good level in Tai Chi; once a week at a class won't get you very far. Confucius said, 'Is it not pleasant to learn with constant perseverance and application?'

It doesn't much matter where or when you practise: the important thing is to put in the time. Yesterday, for example, I did a four-hour seminar and 15 minutes personal training. Today I did eight Neigong exercises with two private students, then gave a private lesson of one hour Sword and one hour Hand Form. It is good to ring the changes, as research has shown that doing the same exercise every day is less beneficial than varying your daily routine.

A problem for most beginners is that they don't know enough form movements to have a worthwhile practice. This book is therefore going to teach you some simple and fun drills.

Tai Chi's a journey, so first work out where you want to go and how soon you want to get there. Be realistic – the moon is far off.

It's also like a bank: the more money (Tai Chi practice) you invest, the more interest (well-being and skill) you earn. The more money you withdraw (booze, smoking and so on), the less capital and interest you'll build up.

If your destination is to improve health, then learning a Hand Form or at least some basic Qigong from a competent tutor and practising it daily is enough to get most folks there.

If you want to go down the martial road and be able to use Tai Chi effectively as a martial art, try to find a tutor who has some real experience of Kung Fu fighting using Tai Chi. There's an urban myth that this practical type of Tai Chi is more difficult to learn than so called 'external' martial arts like Karate. Not true. Good Tai Chi is direct and effective and basic fighting skills can be acquired in a hundred days of practice.

That practice should include a lot of partner work. Pushing Hands drills are essential to develop footwork and body evasion, controlling, striking and locking an opponent at close quarters. You'll also need to practise key applications, many of which are either not named in the form or are entirely separate from the form. As a result few tutors know this stuff. Quite a few of my more senior students get together on a regular basis to practise outside of the classes.

Then you will need to learn some kind of martial Neigong to develop the ability to withstand blows, to strengthen the joints and tendons and stimulate the nervous system.

Some conditioning is a necessity. Since 1975 I've practised punching with a 1.8kg (4lb) weight in each hand, usually a couple of times a week. I do 150 punches a minute for up to 20 minutes. This skill helps to develop one-strike knockdowns. Very few Tai Chi tutors and students have this ability. The weights also help to strengthen the grip, which is useful for Qin Na/Seizing and Holding techniques and for weapons training. We'll discuss conditioning in more depth later (see page 216).

Lastly, if you really want to consider yourself a martial artist, you'll have to learn and practise weapon applications, not just forms.

One of the reasons I became a professional Tai Chi tutor was so I could fit the training in.

Try to vary your training schedule: it should be fun, not a chore. You may also want to prioritize certain skills and not find it necessary to practise other skills quite so much.

Loosening Exercises

It's useful, especially for beginners, to learn some simple loosening exercises that are easy to do and don't take up much space.

Tiger Embraces Head

This is an Inner Form technique: that is, it's hidden inside another technique from the Hand Form. It's mentioned in passing in *The Classic of Boxing*, though it's not one of the official list of 32 techniques found there. Tiger Embraces Head exists in all Yang and Chen lineage Long Forms, though the name has been lost. It occurs just as the arms are crossed and fists are clenched prior to kicking and extending the arms.

Stand in a horse-riding stance, feet about one and a half to two shoulder's widths apart. Flex the knees. 'Stand like a level scale; move like a wheel,' *The Canon of Tai Chi Chuan* advises. We accomplish this by rotating the body on the central axis that extends from the crown of the head to the coccyx. The arms turn and the legs coil one way then the other as we turn the centre line. Do up to 360 of these turns – it should take about 5–6 minutes.

There are quite a few applications of this technique, but a basic one is to sidestep, simultaneously parrying and countering the opponent's attack to the head.

> ### Top tip
> • You can also do the exercise with hand weights, but don't overdo it in terms of exertion or in terms of the size of the weights you use. If in doubt, ask your Tai Chi tutor.

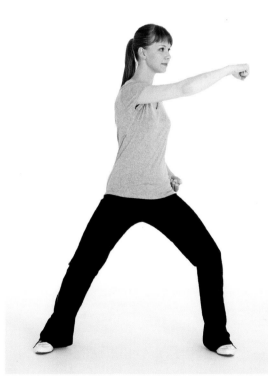

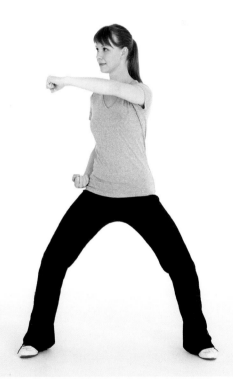

1. Keeping erect in a horse-riding stance, twist the body to the left and punch with the right fist at shoulder level, palm down. Bring the left palm in close to the hip, fist clenched, palm up.

2. Once the whole body is coiled to the left, uncoil by twisting to the right, rotating the central axis as before.

Retrieving the Moon from the Sea

Again, begin in a horse-riding stance. Bend forward until the back is parallel to the ground, arms extended between the legs with the hands palm up; inhale at the same time. Slowly straighten up and bend the torso back, extending the arms up and out from the body. At the same time, exhale. This exercise (see below) is good for flexibility and strengthens the spine and lungs. It also promotes abdominal breathing. Each backbend takes 5–6 seconds. Don't do more than 360: that'll take about 45 minutes.

Body Evasion

When we're in a situation where we can't use footwork to evade an attack, we use body evasion. As previously mentioned, the preferred response when attacked involves moving the feet. Sometimes this can be impossible. In these cases we need to use body evasion: bending back when being attacked to the head and bending in at the waist when attacked to the body. The idea is to make the target unavailable.

Top tip
• When bending back, count to three and bend a little further back with each count.

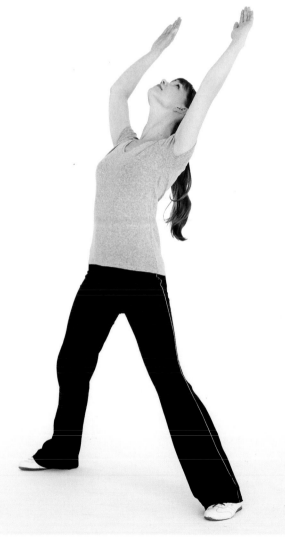

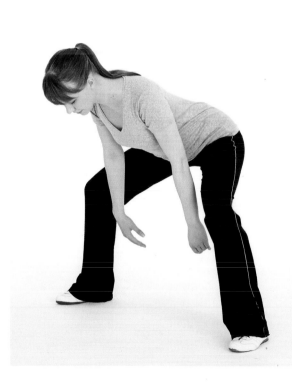

1. In a horse-riding stance, bend forward to stretch and realign the spine; keep the hands palm up, between the legs.

2. Bend backwards and stretch. This exercise is to train flexibility in order to use body evasion, such as swaying back to avoid your opponent's punch.

Bamboo Bending

This is a partnered flexibility drill where each partner in turn plants the feet on the ground in a front stance while the other pulls and pushes him in all directions. The first partner's feet remain rooted to the ground while his body goes with the gentle but continuous pushes and pulls, like bamboo in a strong wind. The aim is to train softness and relaxation and to avoid stiffness. Take it in turns to be the bending bamboo and do at least five minutes each.

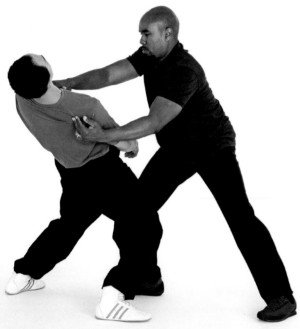

1. Absorb his force by bending backward.

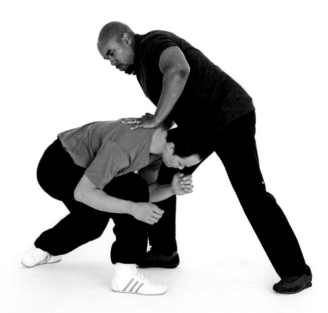

2. Bend forward and don't resist as your opponent presses down on you.

3. Sway back to absorb his pressure.

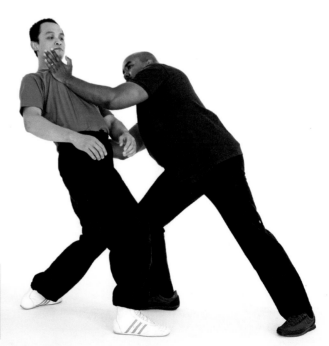

Top tip
• Keep your centre of gravity low as your partner leads your movements.

Tui Shou/Pushing Hands

This form of partnered training is not well understood in many schools. Firstly, there are drills to train harmonizing with a partner's actions, which are also designed to improve coordination and the transfer of body weight. Then there are many footwork drills which train distance timing and angle. Those interested can find more key drills in my book *The Tai Chi Bible*. In terms of application, most Tai Chi practitioners lack the quality of Zou/movement as mentioned in The Tai Chi Chuan Classics. The essence of Zou is to use the feet to evade an attack and to give momentum to your counter. In Tai Chi, as elsewhere, force is made up of mass multiplied by acceleration.

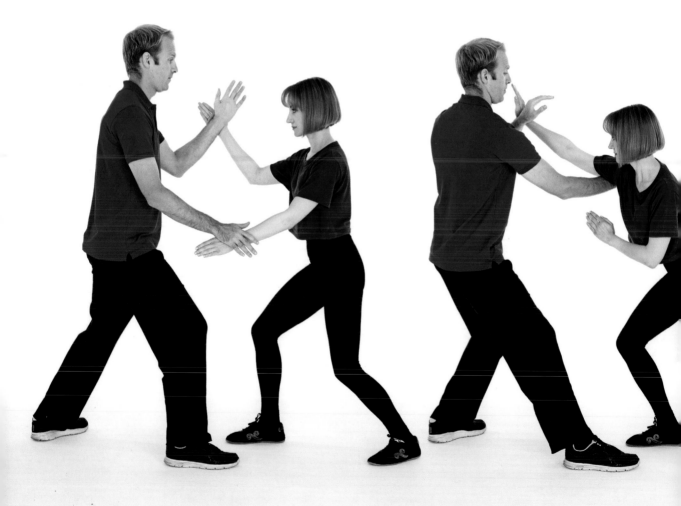

1. Start by making contact with your opponent's arms, so that you can feel what she is doing.

2. When she attempts a push, trap her arm and use it as a lever to uproot her.

聽

Above The Chinese character for Ting.

An Interpretation of the Practice of the 13 Tactics advises, 'Move like a mighty river.' So we need to be continuous, not stopping and starting again.

As well as drills, there is also free pushing, where both partners try to keep their own balance while trying to disrupt the other's. The main skill in free pushing is Ting, which means listening. The Chinese character for this (see left) consists of, at the bottom left, three horizontal and one vertical line; this character means disciple. At the top right there is a cross: this is the number ten. At the upper left, what looks like a ladder is the character for ear. Below the cross are three boxes: the character for eye. At the bottom right is the character for heart/ mind. So we have a disciple who

assiduously (ten times) uses his eyes, ears and mind to listen. In Pushing Hands, through our contact with our opponent we are trying to feel his use of Jin/skilled force. At close distance it is unwise to rely only on the eyes to tell us what is going on; if we wait until the eyes tell the brain what is happening and the brain formulates a response and tells the body what to do, it's often too late. If we have physical contact with the opponent, our listening skills can detect what is happening early on and help to formulate an instant response.

In order to enhance the listening ability, some schools, including my own, sometimes practise certain Pushing Hands drills as well as free Pushing Hands with the eyes shut. A couple of times, I've taught blind folk to do this. They had lots of fun.

In order to control the opponent and to feel his attempted use of Jin, we need to adhere with our arms to his. If we don't adhere, we can't listen or control and it becomes a hitting situation – very dangerous at close quarters. We want to be soft when listening; the term used in The Tai Chi Chuan Classics is Mian, meaning cotton. It's less effort to be soft and it's easier to change from soft to hard than from hard to soft.

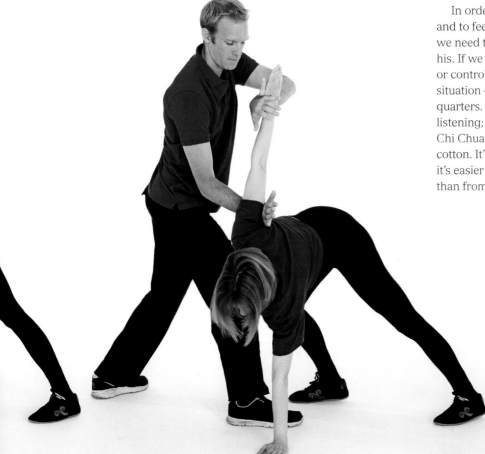

3. She is led into the void and loses balance.

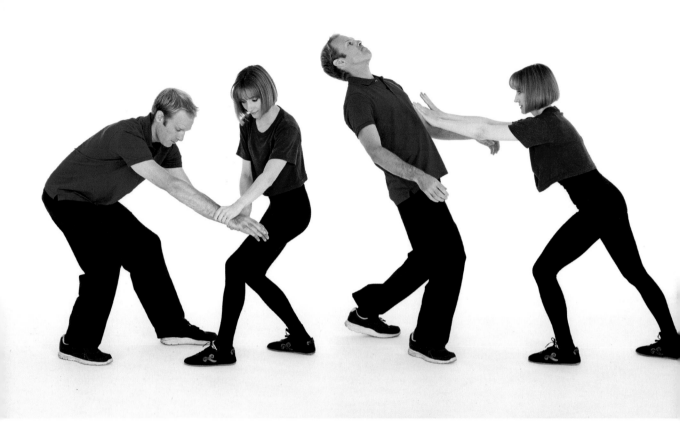

1. When you try to uproot your opponent with a pull, he resists.

2. Add to his force by changing to a push.

If we can feel the opponent's force, we divert or neutralize it; this is called Hua Jin. Hua is to transform, so we use our force to transform the opponent's force. Finally, we discharge skilled force ourselves; this is Fa Jin.

The other main error in Pushing Hands is using force against force, although we can sometimes fool the opponent by pretending to do so.

Pushing Hands is done at close quarters; it represents the point in a fight when we have closed with an opponent. At Pushing Hands distance we should be either striking or trying to control the opponent so that we can unbalance him; we can then either follow up with a strike or try to put a lock on him.

The Fighter's Song intones, 'Entice the opponent into the void, harmonize, then promptly discharge.'

This is telling us to get out of the way of the opponent's attack so that he has nothing to hit. We harmonize our distance, timing and angle with him. This is called Sui/following – often inaccurately translated as 'yielding'. We then counter his attack before he can recover.

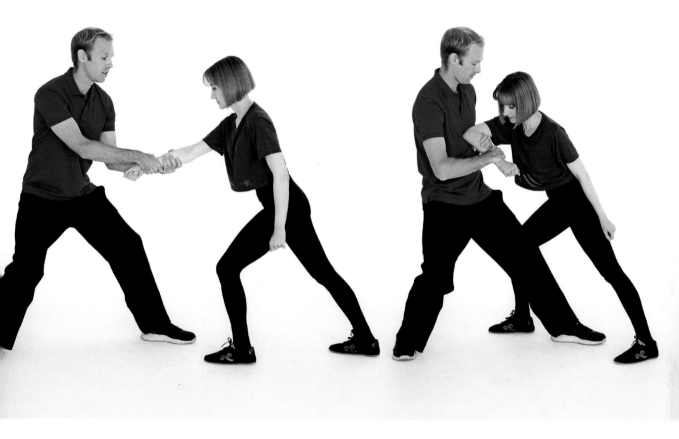

3. He attempts a pull.

4. Go with his force and strike him with your elbow.

The void means more than just emptiness. With correct body mechanics, we can resist a push from a bigger person. With a correct angle of push or pull it is possible for a much smaller person to unbalance a larger one.

This line of least resistance is effectively a diagonal line bisecting the opponent's/partner's stance. It is the key to making a lot of techniques effective.

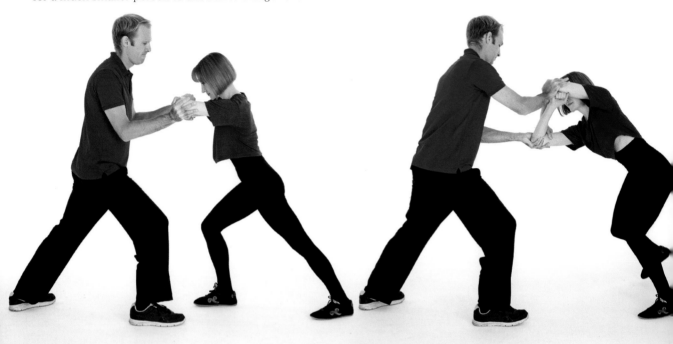

1. If your opponent is well rooted, even if you are bigger and heavier, her body mechanics enable her to resist a direct push. The force of that push goes into the ground.

2. If you push diagonally your opponent will be unable to resist. This angle is the void.

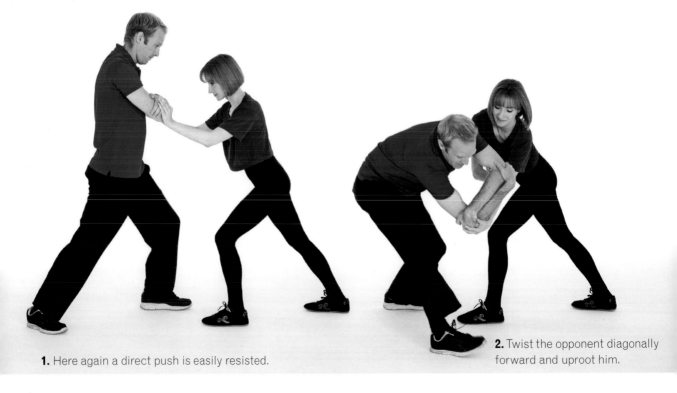

1. Here again a direct push is easily resisted.

2. Twist the opponent diagonally forward and uproot him.

Single-Hand Pushing Hands

This exercise trains you to coordinate the limbs and body weight. Both partners begin with the right foot forward and use the reverse (left) hand to perform the exercise. Put the weight behind the push by transferring it on to the front foot as you push your partner's arm in towards his body. As you do this, he rests his weight forward on that arm, so you have something to push against. Once he turns his hips to the left he continues to turn and diverts your pushing arm to the left also. He then makes his own push by placing the sole of his right foot on the ground to drop his centre of gravity and to be rooted.

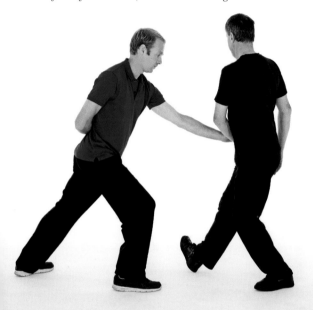

1. The pusher's weight is well forward.

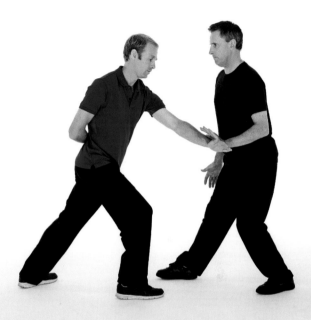

2. The partner's weight is well back so he can absorb the push.

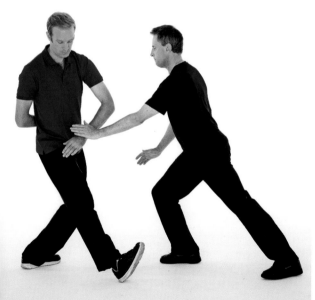

3. The partner diverts the push to his left and then pushes his partner in turn. After 10 minutes, change feet and do the same thing on the other side.

Top tip
• Use the legs and the body, not the arms, to push and divert.

Da Lu/Big Diversion

This advanced Pushing Hands drill seems to exist in all styles of Tai Chi and is generally considered to be the most complex. It's best known as Da Lu, but is more formally known as Four Corners or Eight Gates and Five Steps.

We'll start with the footwork. Both partners have the right foot forward, one in a back stance (Yin), the other in a front stance (Yang). Yang takes a circular step, around to the left and towards Yin, who takes a step back with the right foot. Yang takes two more steps forward, right then left, ending up in a back stance. Yin responds, stepping back with the left foot then across with the right foot into a front stance. They match the timing of their steps. The same process is now repeated back the other way. After the moves become fluent, repeat the drill, starting with left foot forward.

This drill involves four of the Eight Forces: uproot/ Cai, spiral/Lie, forearm/Zhou and barge/Kao. The angle of application is seen as being diagonal, hence the name Four Corners.

The aim of Da Lu is to use the opponent's hands and arms as levers with which to unbalance and manipulate him, and to counter using footwork when he tries to do this to you. Maintain the distance, match the timing, use correct footwork.

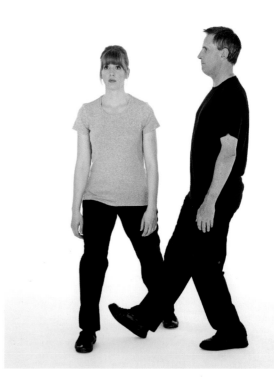

1. Begin in a front stance (like the lady in this sequence), right foot forward. Your partner is in a back stance, also with the right foot forward, at a right angle to you.

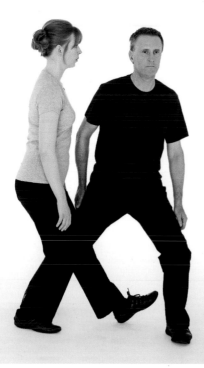

4. Move into a back stance with your left foot while he turns into a front stance, left foot forward.

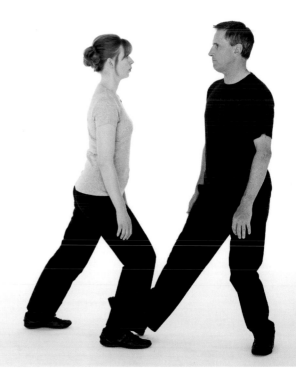

5. As your partner steps around to the right with his back foot, step back with your left foot.

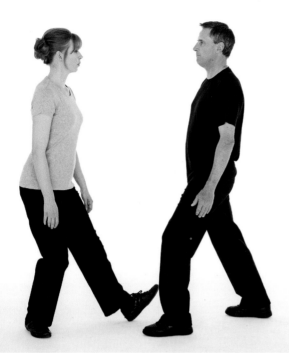

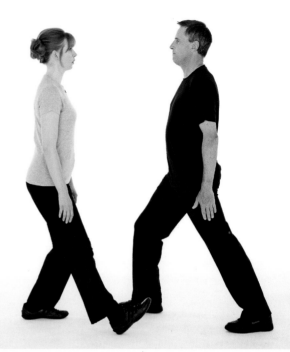

2. Step around to the left with your back foot, while he steps back with his right foot.

3. Step forward with your right foot, while he steps back with his left foot.

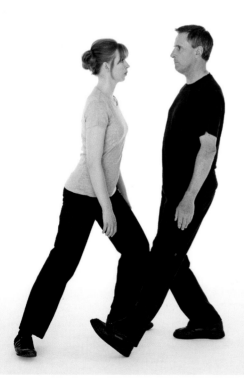

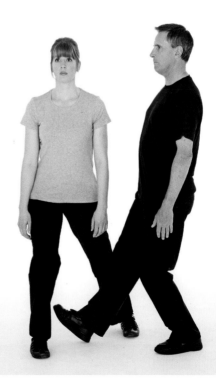

6. When he steps forward with his left foot, match him by stepping back with your right foot.

7. As he takes another step with his right foot, step into a front stance again, right foot forward. You are now back where you started.

Now we add the arm movements. Yang grasps Yin's right wrist with the right hand and uses the left forearm (Zhou) to lock Yin's upper arm. Yin attempts to barge (Kao) Yang with the right shoulder. Yin presses and pulls down suddenly to uproot (Cai) Yang, who spirals (Lie) the force round and into Zhou again. You then repeat with the roles reversed. When you are both fluent, Yang starts with the Zhou on Yin's left arm and the whole process begins again.

Next we combine and coordinate arm and foot movements as shown. The footwork later becomes more complex and we learn to visit all Eight Gates/directions in turn, applying the Four Corner forces. We also learn how to instantaneously reverse roles and change directions.

The essence of Da Lu is summed up in *An Interpretation of the Practice of the 13 Tactics*:

'The steps follow the changes of the body…
Moving back and forth, there must be turning over and folding up.
In advancing and retreating, there must be turning a
nd change.'

In doing this, we adhere. We are soft. We are continuous. We follow. We don't lose contact or use force against force.

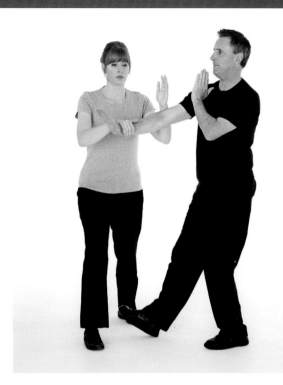

1. Begin in a front stance, right foot forward. Your partner is in a back stance, also with his right foot forward, at a right angle to you. Control him using your forearm/Zhou to apply a lock to his right arm. Because you are in control, you are said to be in the Yang position, while he is in the Yin.

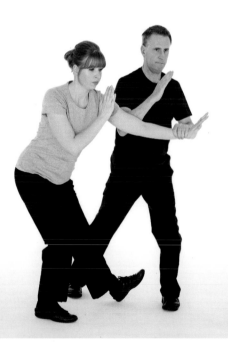

4. Move into a back stance with your left foot while he turns into a front stance, left foot forward, locking your left arm with his forearm (Zhou).

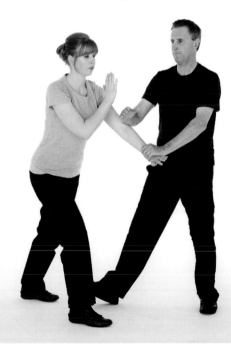

5. To prevent you barging him (Kao), he presses down on your left arm to uproot you (Cai). At the same time, he steps around to the right with his back foot, while you step back with your left foot.

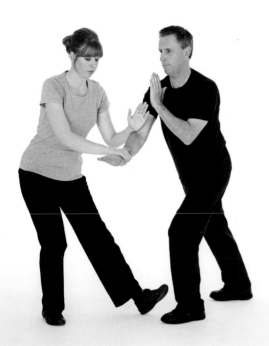

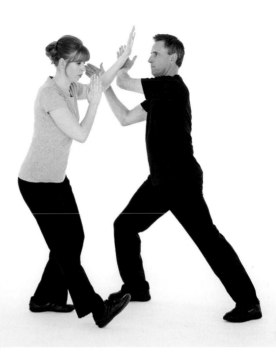

2. To prevent your partner from barging you (using Kao), press down on his right arm to uproot him (Cai). At the same time, step around to the left with your back foot, while he steps back with his right foot.

3. Step forward with your right foot, while your partner steps back with his left foot, using a spiralling force (Lie) on your left arm.

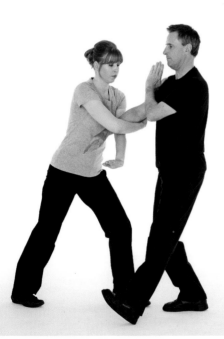

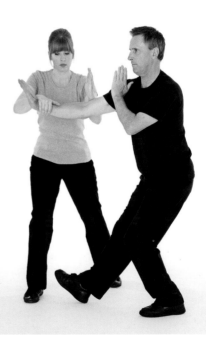

6. Step back with your right foot, while your partner steps forward with his left foot. At the same time use a spiralling force (Lie) on his left arm.

7. Turn into a front stance with the right foot forward as before, locking his left arm with your forearm (Zhou) as he steps forward with the right foot into a back stance. You are now back where you started.

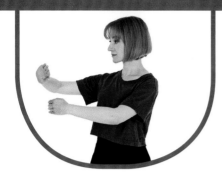

Hand Form

In the Wu lineage, Wu Jianquan is credited with inventing the Square Form, a deconstructed, simplified method for beginners; once they have learned this they move on to learning the traditional Round Form. The idea is to give beginners the structure and then to build technique on to it.

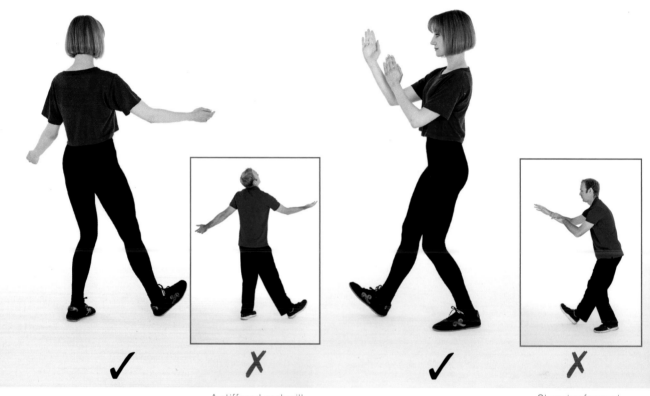

✔   ✘

A stiffened neck will force the neck, back and body out of alignment.

✔   ✘

Slumping forward.

1. Xu Ling Ding Jin/Empty the headtop and neck of strength This is an instruction which appears in *The Canon of Tai Chi Chuan*. We relax the neck and align the headtop with the spine. If there is stiffness in the head and neck, it affects the Jingshen/vigour and leads to clumsiness. The head and neck should be free from tension; they go easily with the force as we apply it. Note that when the head is attacked, taking it out of alignment can be the most sensible thing to do. Training forms without breaking head/neck alignment also help us to develop peripheral vision.

2. Hollow the chest to raise the back This advice is often misunderstood: it does not mean hunch over and collapse the chest. Unfortunately some Tai Chi schools have taken their practice to an extreme, which has sometimes led to practitioners becoming somewhat hunchbacked. Yang Chengfu is saying, 'Don't push out the chest or you'll become top heavy – it'll also cause compression on the discs and vertebrae and prevent abdominal breathing. Keep your upper body correctly aligned; be straight without being stiff.'

In 30 years of knowing him, I never saw my teacher do the complete Long Hand Form all the way through from beginning to end, although he taught form regularly. His forms were 70–80 per cent the same as the Wu Jianquan lineage, but the Spear was almost entirely different.

Yang Chengfu, the person most responsible for Tai Chi's worldwide popularity, is also famous for his ten important points regarding Tai Chi practice, which he is supposed to have dictated to his student, Chen Weiming. For a big, fat guy weighing more than 135kg (300lb), his Tai Chi photos show that his postures and stance work were excellent. There's a lot more to Tai Chi theory than what is contained in these ten points and they are often misinterpreted anyway, but they are a useful shorthand guide to better practice. Allow me to reinterpret the ten points for you.

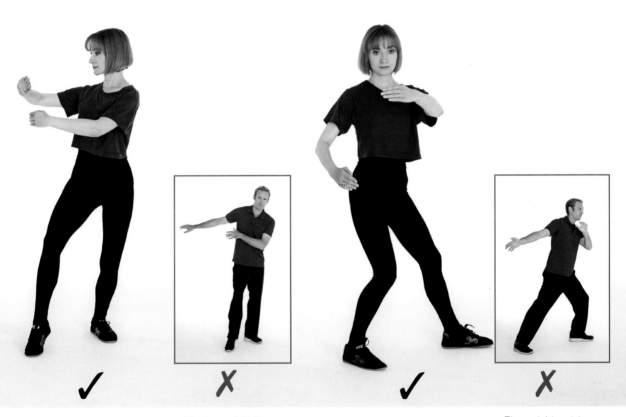

✔ ✘

Moving mainly the arms, but not the body.

✔ ✘

The weight arriving before the technique, rather than with it.

3. Relax the waist This doesn't just mean turn the waist and hips. Yang is telling us to relax and let the centre line turn in accordance with the technique being performed (rotating and flexing the spine as in tennis, golf and many other activities, not just Tai Chi). Shifting your weight comes with this centre-line rotation. *An Interpretation of the Practice of the 13 Tactics* also advises us, 'The strength comes from the spine.'

4. Clearly distinguish void/empty and substantial/ full In addition to practising your form, you need to practise Pushing Hands drills and applications to be spontaneously able to change your position and weight distribution in accordance with the technique you are applying. Many Tai Chi practitioners think that this advice relates only to the feet and that one foot should be full of weight at all times, while the other should be void/empty of weight. They are wrong on both counts.

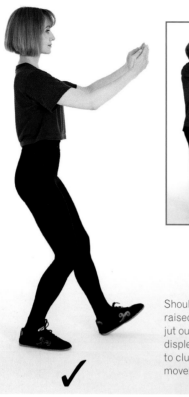

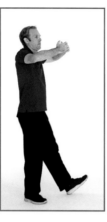

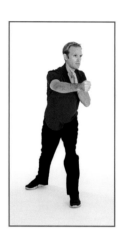

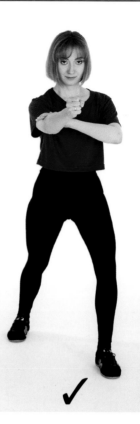

Shoulders are raised and elbows jut out. Aesthetically displeasing leading to clumsy, jerky movements.

Use of force is a bit excessive, resulting in over-extension and incorrect alignment.

5. Sink the shoulders and lower the elbows If your shoulders are raised and your elbows jut out, your arms and centre line become stiff, leading to jerky movements. This admonition is sometimes misinterpreted as advising minimal arm extension when pushing and striking as in Brush Knee Twist Step or Deflect, Parry and Punch. Old Tai Chi form photos of Yang Chengfu show the big man to have had large expansive postures; I like his approach, being a reasonably big guy myself.

6. Use the Yi/intention and not Li/physical strength In *The Song of the 13 Tactics*, we chant, 'The principle is to use the intent' and 'The Yi and the Qi are the rulers.' From *An Interpretation of the Practice of the 13 Tactics*, we quote, 'The body and the Yi are entirely concentrated on the Jingshen/vigour, not on the Qi. If on the Qi, there is stagnation.' The movements control the breath in Tai Chi. They should be done with intent so that they become purposeful and smooth; knowing the martial applications of each technique is of great help in this process.

7. 'Above and below accompany one another' is another quotation from *The Fighter's Song*. It refers there to the use of force. *The Tai Chi Chuan Discourse* tells us, 'If there's up, there's down.' We use total body force and apply circular force on the opponent; if there is resistance we simply reverse the direction in which we are applying force. From above to below, the whole body must be coordinated and able to change.

His opponent presses him forward and down, but he resists.

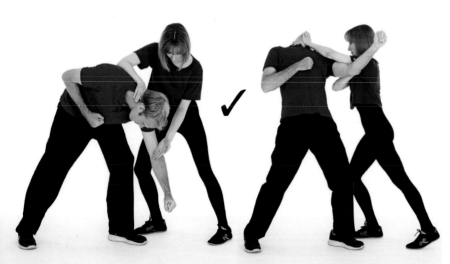

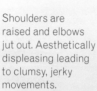

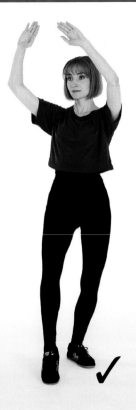

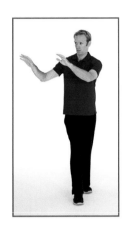

Hands are too low,
so the movement
is less effective in
working the breath
and circulation.

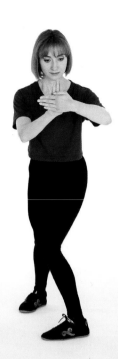

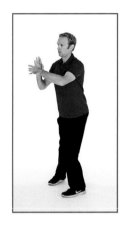

Moving into the next
movement without
completing the
previous one.

8. Internal and external in cooperation The use of the
spine and the movements of the limbs control the breath
and stimulate the Three Treasures of Qi, Jing and Shen
(see pages 80–1). These movements in turn are controlled
by Yi/intent.

9. Continuity of movement without breaking off
The movements of the form should be smooth and continuous,
not jerky or ending abruptly. The difficulty is still to make
the movements clearly defined. There are a lot of Tai Chi
people around whose techniques lack definition.

10. Seek stillness in movement
The Song of the 13 Tactics tells us, 'There is stillness
even when there is movement. In movement yet there is
stillness.' When we are moving, the mind is still, in the
sense of calm. When training static postures yet there
is circulation and movement of the internal organs – in
Taoist terminology, there is a oneness.

Weapons

The classical weapons of Chinese martial arts are Qiang/Spear, Dao/Sabre or Broadsword and Jian/Straight Sword. The use of these three weapons in forms and in application is traditionally part of the Tai Chi syllabus.

The Spear and the Sword are identified with the dragon, so the emphasis is on soaring and plunging with sudden thrusts. The Sabre is identified with the tiger, so the stances are long and low. There is much crouching, much leaping and much slashing.

My own Sifu didn't like Tai Chi Sword much, preferring the directness of Spear and Sabre. When I came to develop my own method I had to change some weapon applications, as techniques I found in my European medieval and renaissance Sword manuals were often more effective than those he'd shown me.

Tai Chi weapon techniques can be adapted for use with everyday objects, such as sticks, umbrellas and so on. But it's a lot of fun to practise with weapons. Besides, you can't really consider yourself to be a proper martial artist unless you can use weapons.

For a fuller discussion of weapon training, see my book *The Tai Chi Bible*.

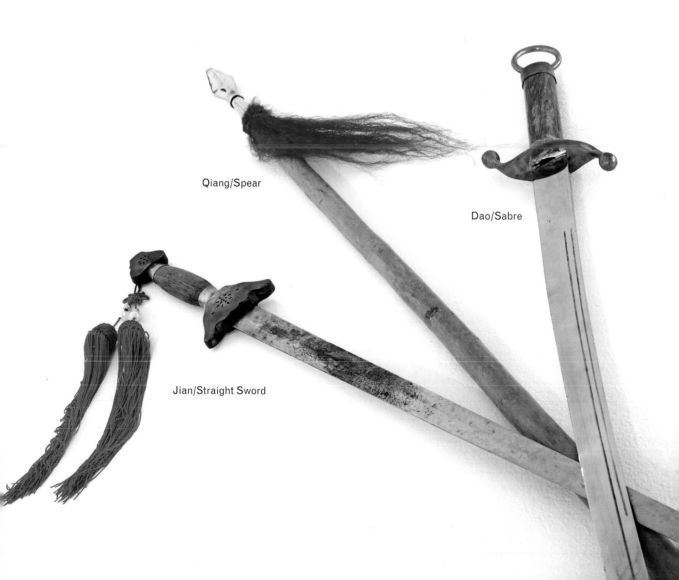

Qiang/Spear

Dao/Sabre

Jian/Straight Sword

Neigong

This term is often translated as internal strength. In Wu lineage there is a Neigong tradition of 24 exercises. In some schools, such as my Sifu's, these exercises are separated into 12 Yin and 12 Yang sequences with a precise training pattern for each exercise. In other schools, such as the Wu family, there is no such division.

Most of the exercises have martial applications and include internal alchemy, meditative and therapeutic aspects, as well as basic strengthening. These exercises, too, are part of a lost Tai Chi, because few people practise them. This is mainly because they are physically demanding and time-consuming. There's also a ceremony of discipleship involved before the exercises can be taught.

On a personal level I do Neigong every day. As with anything else, if you want to learn this aspect of Tai Chi you need a good tutor; incorrect Neigong practice can be physically and mentally damaging. Over the years I've done quite a bit of remedial Neigong tuition.

My late chum Luk Siu-sun was a White Crane boxer who trained in Tai Chi in Hong Kong with my Sifu's uncle and then with my Sifu. He was a big, bluff and hearty chap who was fun to be around, but he'd learned only 16 of the 24 Neigong exercises.

Luk published a book on Tai Chi after relocating to North America. His form technique photos are so appalling, it's as if he set out to defy every criteria from The Tai Chi Chuan Classics. But the book also includes photos of him taking punches to his large gut (he always folded his arms, so his solar plexus and ribs were protected); he even has a photo of himself posing with Muhammad Ali. He'd challenge people to donate money to charity in return for the right to punch. He became famous for this in many Chinese communities.

One day my Sifu got a phone call from a man who taught Yang-style Tai Chi in San Francisco. The man said he'd learned my Sifu's Neigong and knew we could take people jumping onto the abdomen from head height. He said that at a martial arts event he'd got one of his students to do the jump on him from high on a ladder. He'd hurt himself very badly and was passing and coughing up blood. Sifu asked the man who'd taught him the Neigong. It was our old friend Luk Siu-sun.

My Sifu sent the man to relearn and practise the 12 Yin exercises from an old student who worked as a garbage collector in San Francisco's Chinatown. This cured him.

Caveat emptor.

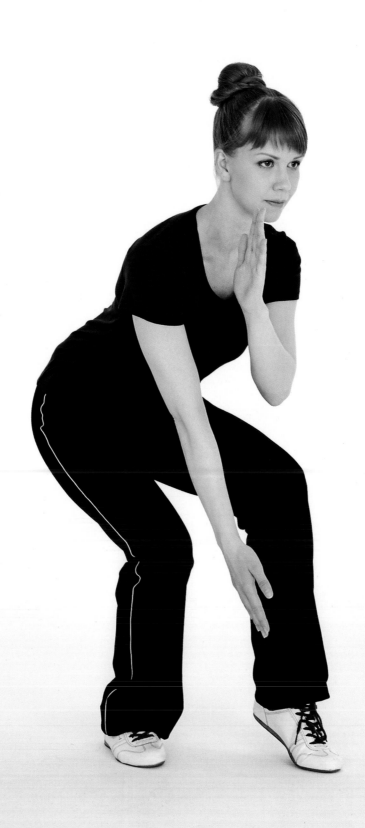

7 The 48 Techniques

The 48 techniques illustrated in this chapter appear in this sequence (with all repetitions omitted) in the Long Form which I teach, and the vast majority of these techniques, or variations thereof, can be found in every Yang lineage Long Form. What is demonstrated here is not a form as such, but is mainly for comparison purposes.

Although the following techniques are demonstrated on one side of the body only, in form and in application they should be practised on both sides of the body. The photos at the top of the page are there as a guide to what your Tai Chi tutor advises you to focus on.

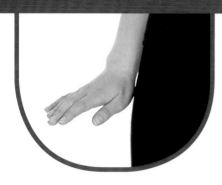

1 Wu Chi

Tai Chi at Rest

This preparatory position concentrates body and spirit prior to doing the form.

1. Stand with the feet a shoulder's width apart and slightly turned out. The palms should be parallel to the ground. The feet should feel rooted to the ground; the spine should be erect.

Top tip

• The arms and legs are straight, but don't lock the joints or the movements will be stiff.

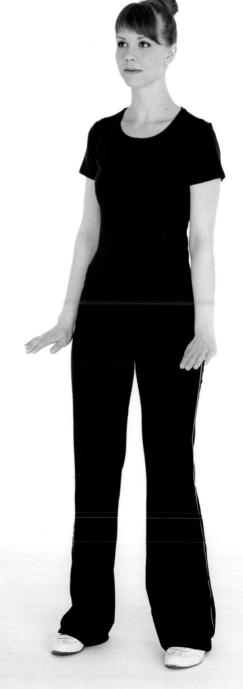

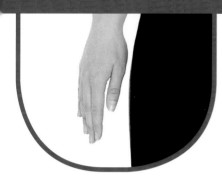

2 Tai Chi

Ready Style

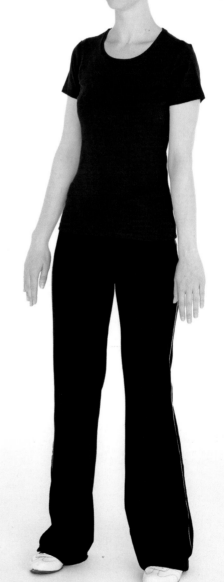

1. This preparatory position is the same as Wu Chi, except the fingers now point down.

Top tip
• Maintain soft hands.

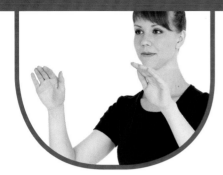

3 Beginning Style

Top tip
• Focus on coordinating arms and legs.

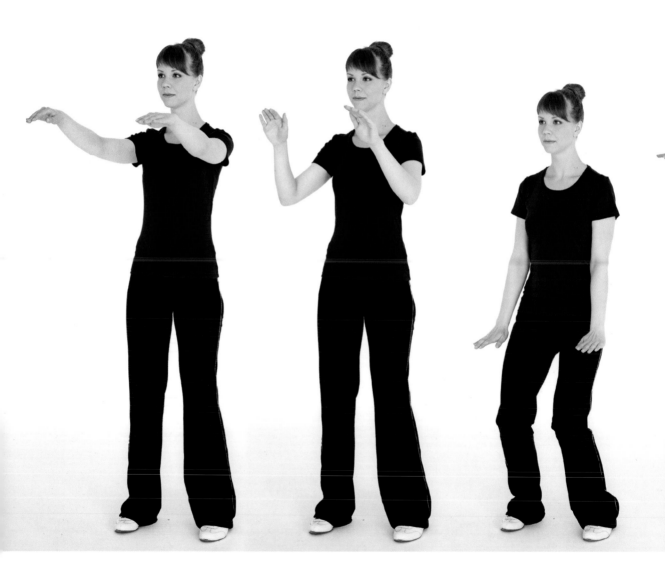

1. Slowly raise the arms to shoulder height.

2. Bend the elbows and inhale as you bring the arms in towards the body; at the same time open the rib cage.

3. Bend the knees, sink, exhale, close the rib cage and lower the arms.

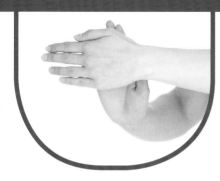

4 Vanguard Arms and Extending Arms

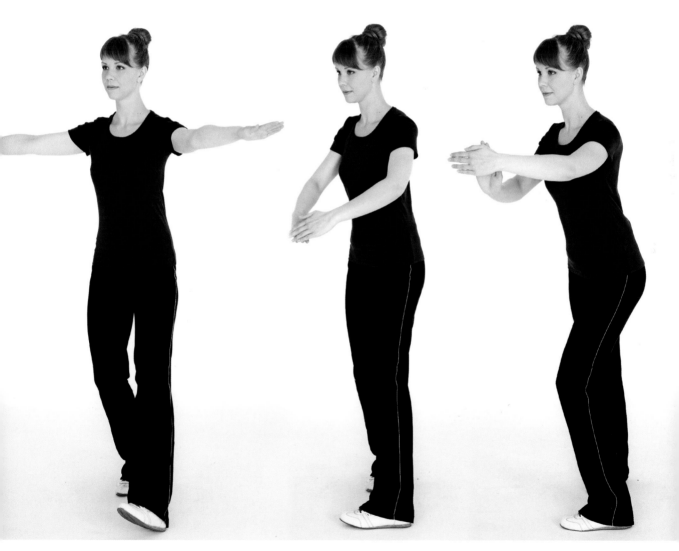

1. Extend the arms out and up to shoulder level, and step forward with the left foot.

2. As you bring the arms in towards the centre, turn the left foot in.

3. Bring the hands up in front of the chest, palm facing palm, and at the same time shift the weight onto the left foot. Incline your body weight forwards into the technique.

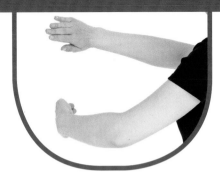

5 Seven Stars Style

Some styles call this position Stroke the Lute; indeed the two techniques are very similar. The seven stars are represented by the shoulders, elbows and wrists and the fingertips of the front hand.

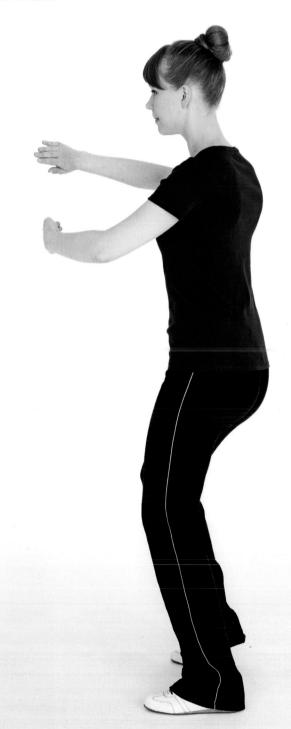

1. Following on from the previous technique, turn right by pivoting on the ball of the rear foot, simultaneously reaching over with the right hand. This trains spinal rotation and focus.

Top tip

- It is mainly the body that is moving, not the arms.

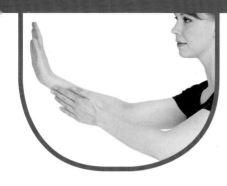

6 Grasping Bird's Tail

In this technique we use Four of the Eight Forces, namely Peng/upward force, Lu/sideways diversion, Ji/push and An/downward press.

Top tip
• Use the body, not the arms.

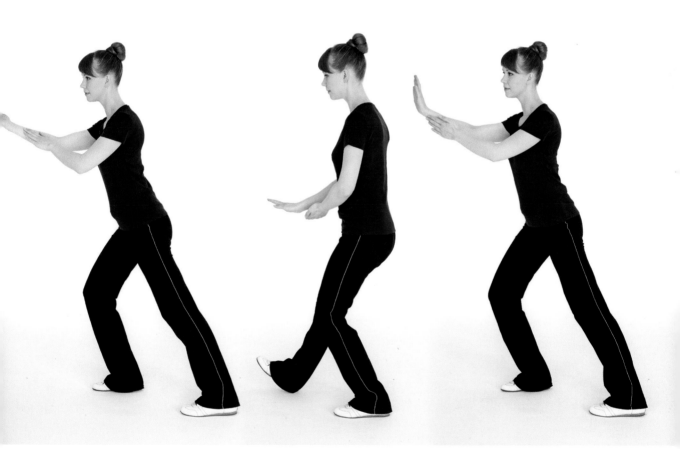

1. Following on from the previous technique, bring the body and arms around to the right; turn both arms as you bring them under and then up to the right as you step forward on to the right foot. This is Peng.

2. Turn the body to the right and start to bring the weight back, turning the arms. This is Lu. Bring the hands in to the left hip. This is An.

3. Shift the weight forward and push out at 45 degrees with the right palm. This is Ji.

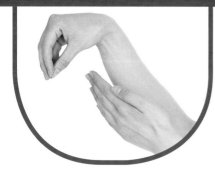

7 Single Whip

This is a technique common to all Tai Chi Chuan styles, though there are considerable variations in execution. In the Wu Quanyou lineage, to which I belong, the technique is executed in a horse-riding stance when it is performed in Hand Form. It is also one of the most repeated techniques in the Long Form (it occurs more than ten times in the form I practice), which gives a hint as to its relative importance. When talking of Single Whip, many exponents tend to think of the completed position, but at its most sophisticated there is much coiling and uncoiling of arms, legs and torso before arriving at that point.

Top tip
• In a horse-riding stance, stand with the feet about two shoulder widths apart.

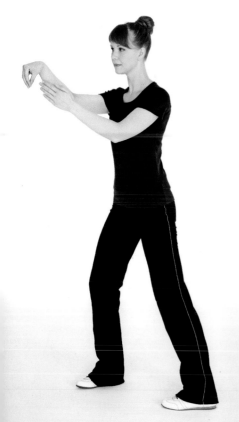

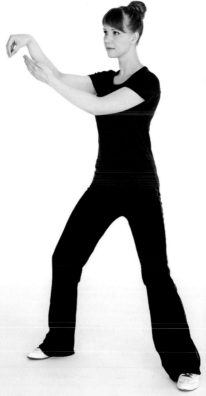

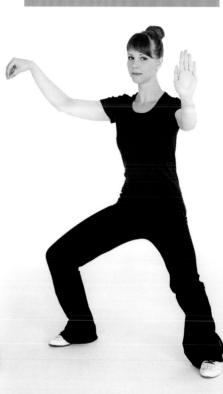

1. Following on from the previous technique; keep the right arm extended, turn the body and turn the front foot in slightly, bringing the right arm around to the left in an arc, at the end of which the right hand forms a hook.

2. Step across with the left foot into a horse-riding stance.

3. Bring the left hand across, palm facing in. As it passes the body, turn the left hand then push out and sink.

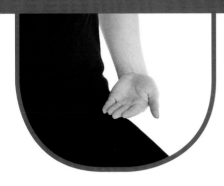

8 Flying Oblique

Flying Oblique can be low or high. Here we demonstrate the high position.

Top tip
• We contract, then expand the body.

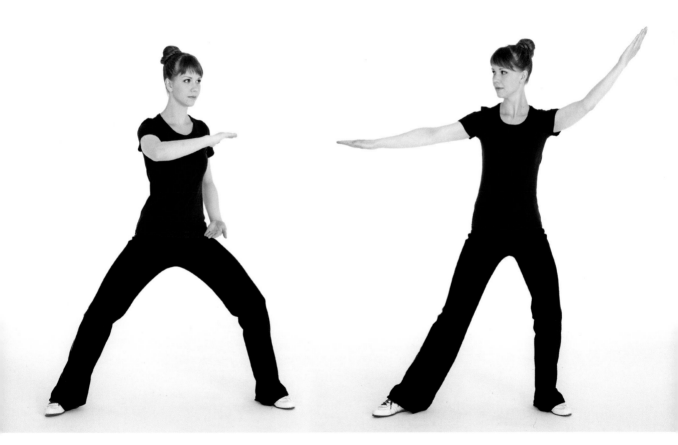

1. Following on from the previous technique; twist the body to the left, bringing the hands into the chest in anti-clockwise circles.

2. Pivot on the right foot and shift the weight on to the left foot, extending the arms. This technique manipulates the limbs by twisting the spine.

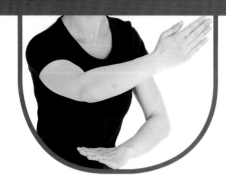

9 Single and Double Hand Seize Legs

These techniques are two Inner Form techniques, but their names are not commonly found in Tai Chi books. They are usually included as part of the following technique, Raise Hands Step Up.

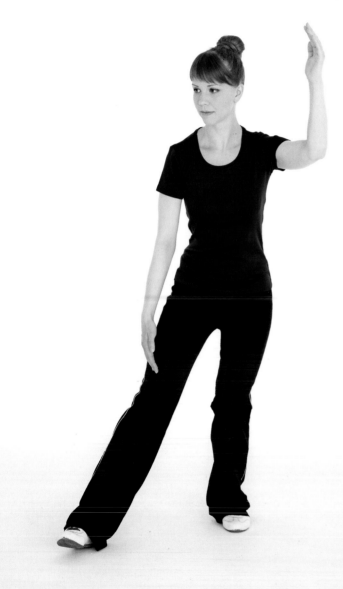

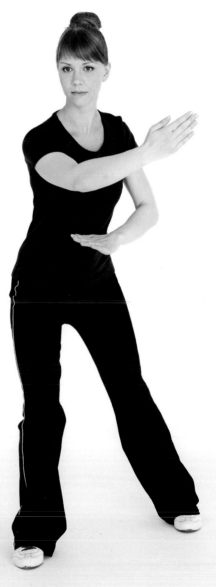

1. Step up with the right foot

2. Start drawing a pair of intersecting circles with the arms. These techniques work on the limbs and spine, while gravity works on the circulation in the arms.

Top tip
• Start off in a low position with the knees bent and stay low.

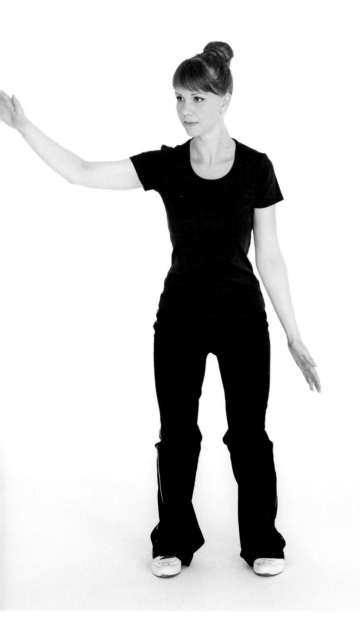

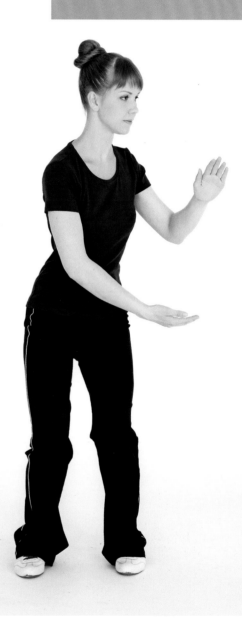

3. Bring the feet together a shoulder's width apart and bend the knes. Make the circles large.

4. The arms should intersect again.

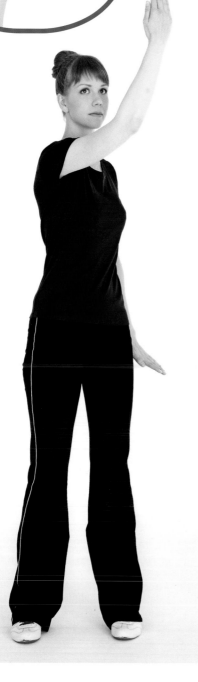

10 Raise Hands Step Up

This technique stretches the whole body including the lungs.

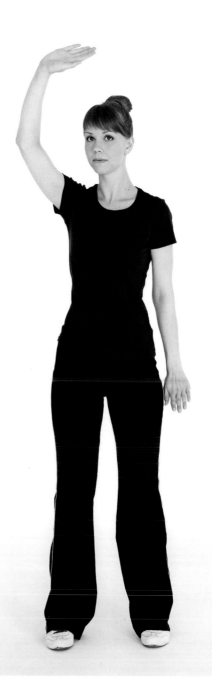

1. Start from Double Hand Seize Legs (see pages 120–1) in a crouched position, with palm facing palm in front of the chest. Straighten both legs and both arms (one up, one down) simultaneously.

2. Turn to face the front. The right arm should twist as you raise it, at the same time the body turns.

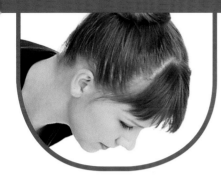

11 White Crane Flaps its Wings

Top tip
• Keep the back straight and don't bend the knees.

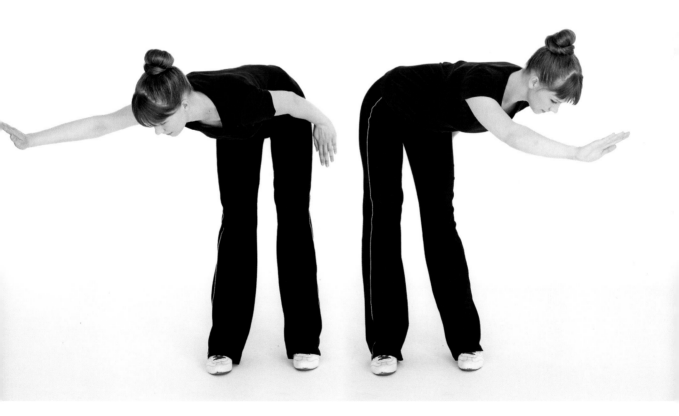

1. Following on from the previous technique, keep the arms in position, bend forward till the torso is about parallel to the ground.

2. Turn the body to the left. This stretches the spinal column and promotes abdominal breathing.

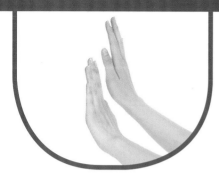

12 Break Arm Style

This is another Inner Form technique, usually considered part of White Crane Flaps its Wings. This technique twists and coils the whole body while also working on the circulation.

Top tip
- Let the body movement lead the arm movement.

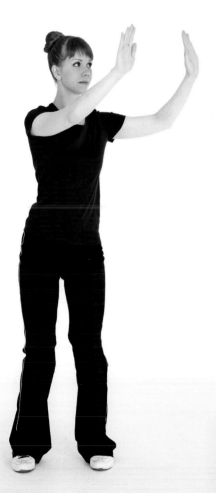

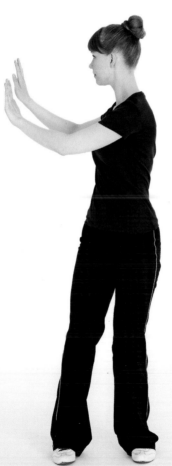

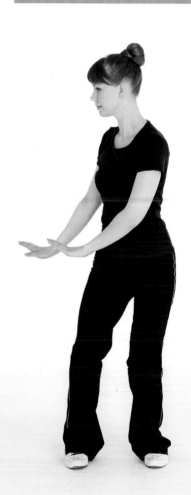

1. Raise both arms and the torso.

2. Turn right.

3. Bring both hands across, high and to the right and then down, at the same time sinking.

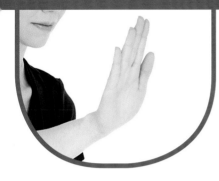

13 Brush Knee Twist Step

Brush Knee Twist Step is so called because in application we brush aside the opponent's kick or catch it in a scooping action with the wrist or elbow joint of our front arm, while giving him a palm strike with our other hand, thus twisting his step and causing him to fall. This would normally be done with a side-step – a movement absent from this form. The transfer forward of the body weight and the palm strike must be coordinated; the finished hand positions are said to resemble the paddling flippers of a terrapin. Brush Knee Twist Step is one of the most repeated and therefore one of the most important techniques in Yang lineage Long Forms.

Top tip

• The weight and the spinal column should be behind the palm strike.

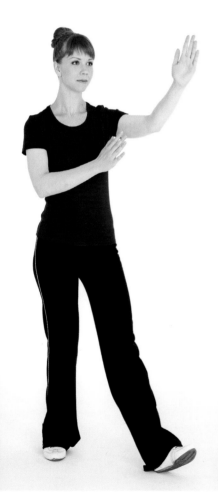

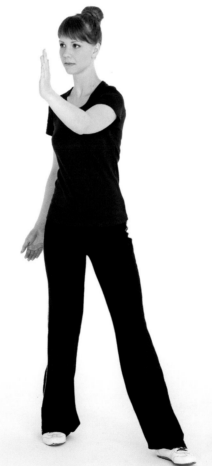

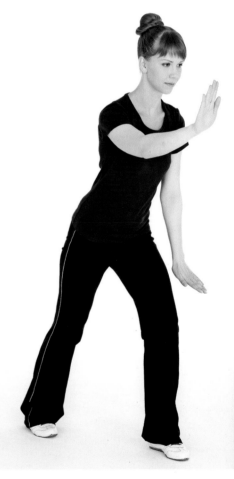

1. Following on from the previous technique, sweeping the arms out to the left, stepping out on to the left heel.

2. The left arm draws a large clockwise circle in front of the body while the right arm draws an anti-clockwise circle to the right.

3. As the right hand finishes its circle with a palm strike, the left hand comes to rest on the outside of the left knee.

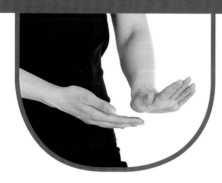

14 Stroke the Lute

Top tip
• The palms face opposite directions throughout the sequence.

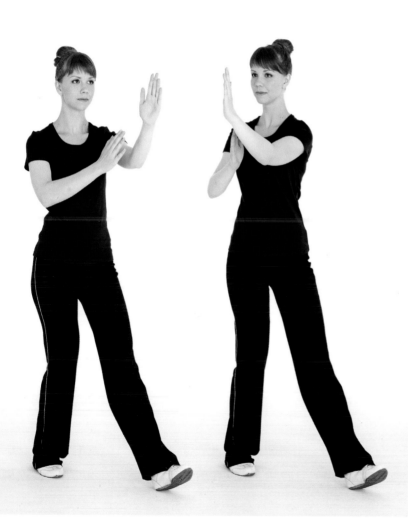

1. Step on to the left heel, with the left hand forward in the Seven Stars position.

2. Turn to the right.

3. Flatten the hands.

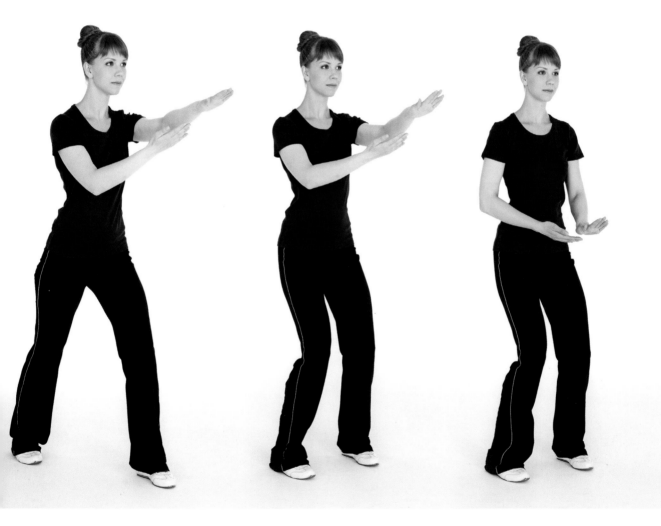

4. Draw an anti-clockwise circle to the left and bring the weight forward.

5. Draw another circle and step up with the back foot so that the feet are a shoulder's width apart.

6. The hands end up in front of the waist.

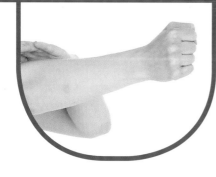

15 Deflect, Parry and Punch

This technique can be done stepping forward or stepping back.

Top tip
• Use the whole body when deflecting and parrying.

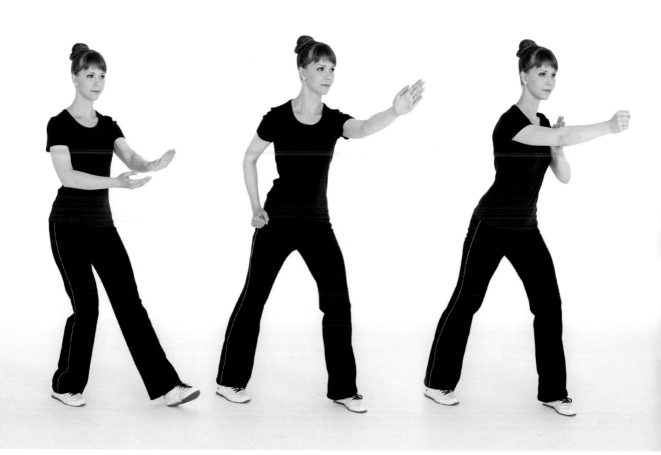

1. Step forward on to the left heel.

2. Extend the left hand, and take the right fist back to the hip.

3. Retract the left hand and extend the right fist.

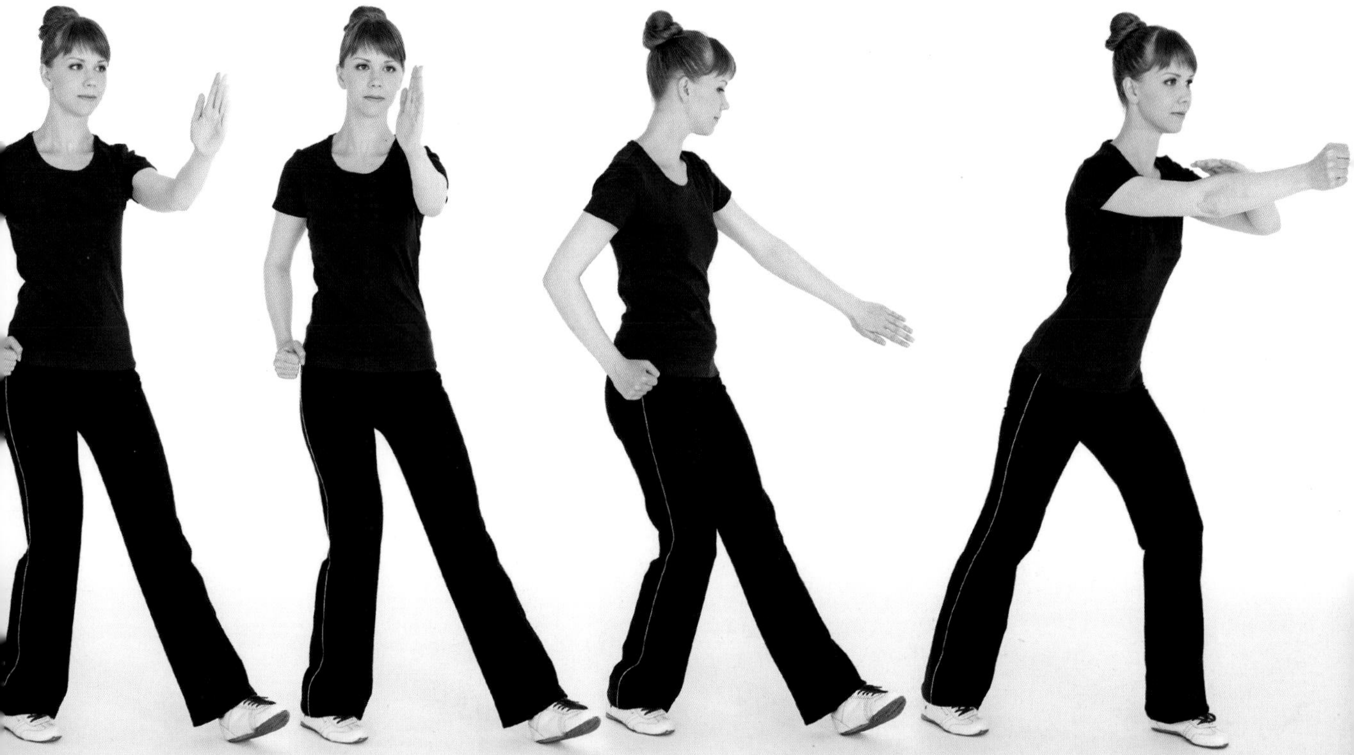

4. Bring the weight back and take the fist back to the hip.

5. Turn the body to the right, bringing the left palm across; this is ban, to remove/deflect (the same term occurs in *The Classic of Boxing*).

6. Now turn to the left and bring the left arm down in a parry; this is Lan.

7. Finally, punch straight ahead with the right fist sliding the left hand to the elbow joint.

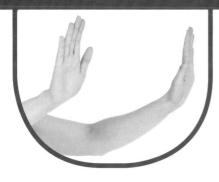

16 As if Shutting a Door

Top tip
• The weight goes forward behind the push, not before it.

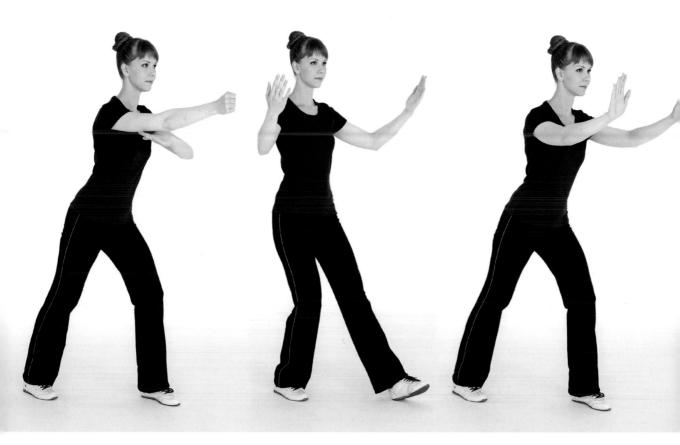

1. Following on from the previous technique, slide the back of the left hand along the underside of the right arm.

2. Bring the weight back and breath in at the same time; move the palms to face towards the body.

3. Shift the weight forward, thrusting from the back leg and pushing with both hands. Breathe out on the push.

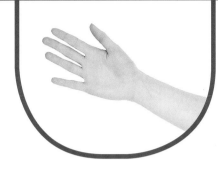

17 Embrace Tiger, Return to Mountain

Top tip
• Keep the arms and legs moving together.

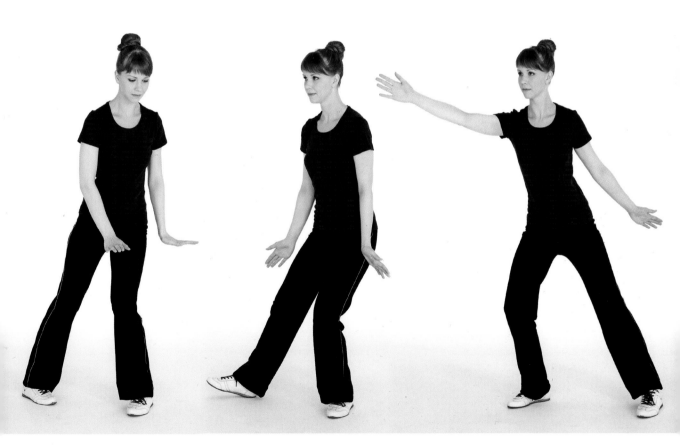

1. Following on from the previous technique, lower the hands, palms down, and, keeping the weight forward, turn the front foot in on the heel.

2. Turn through 135 degrees on the heel of the back foot, turning the arms so the palms face out.

3. Shift the weight onto the right foot and raise the arms, straightening the back leg.

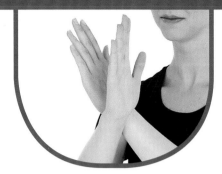

18 Cross Hands

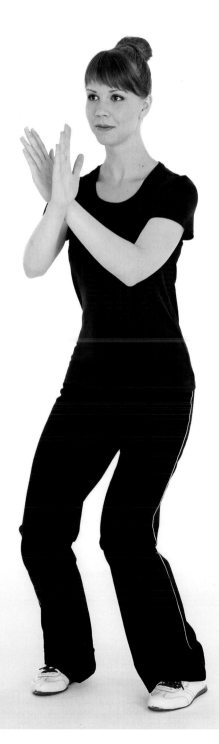

1. Step in with the back foot, keeping the knees bent, and cross the hands in front of the chest.

Top tip
- The arms should not be raised above shoulder level when doing the technique; in application it is a different story.

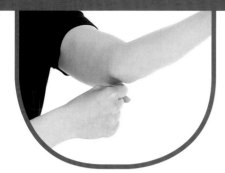

19 Fist Under Elbow

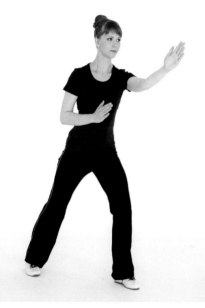

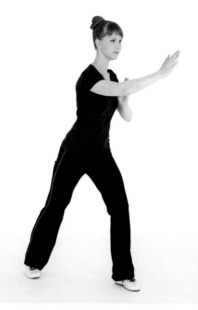

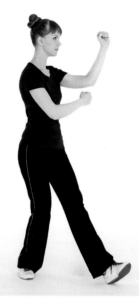

1. Following on from the previous technique, turn the left foot out on the heel and reach to the left with the left hand.

2. Reach over with the right arm.

3. As you shift the weight onto the back foot, make fists (right fist under left elbow) and twist body and limbs left.

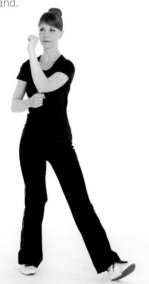

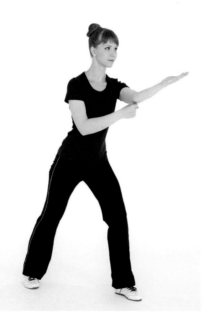

Top tip

• Work on your timing. Many students don't know when to make a fist and when to open a fist.

4. Twist right.

5. Shift the weight forward, opening the left fist as you turn the body to the left. The Chinese term 'zhou di kan chui' literally means 'Under Elbow See Fist'; the opponent sees our fist under his elbow.

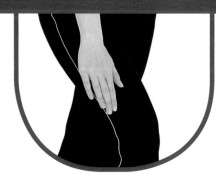

20 Step Back Repulse Monkey

Top tip

• The palm strike and the placing of the left foot on the ground should be simultaneous.

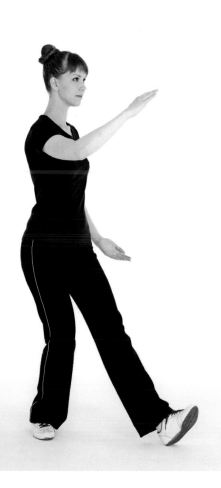

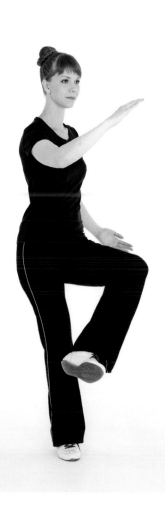

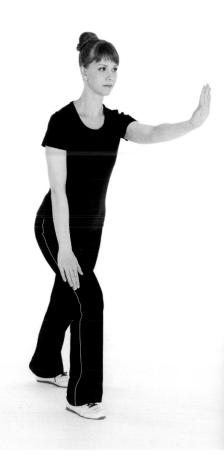

1. Following on from the previous technique, shift into a back stance, turning the body left, and circle the arms clockwise.

2. Raise the front foot with the sole turned in.

3. Step back giving a palm strike. The final position is the same as in Brush Knee Twist Step.

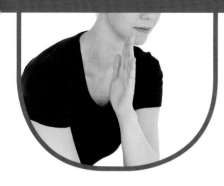

21 Needle at Sea Bottom

Top tip
• Keep the back straight even when inclining forward.

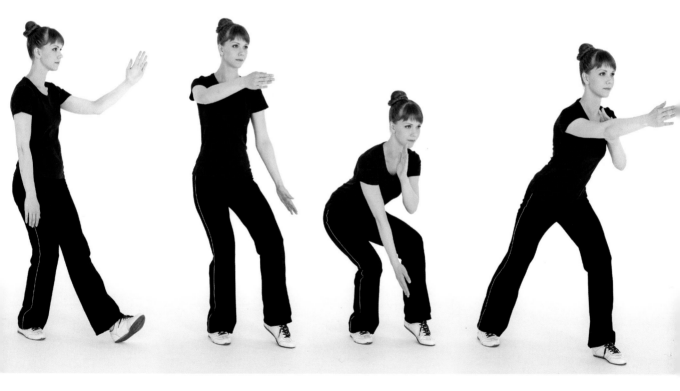

1. Step forward with the left foot, bringing the left hand up to protect the face.

2. Bring the right hand up in an arc. At the same time retract the left foot back onto the ball.

3. Sink and thrust down with the right hand; the left hand protects the face.

4. Step forward with the left foot into a front stance. Bring the right arm up to shoulder level.

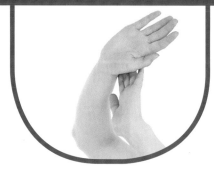

22 Fan Through the Back

Fan Through the Back is the most popular of a variety of names for this technique; the arm movements resemble a fan opening out.

Top tip
- Everything starts and finishes at the same time.

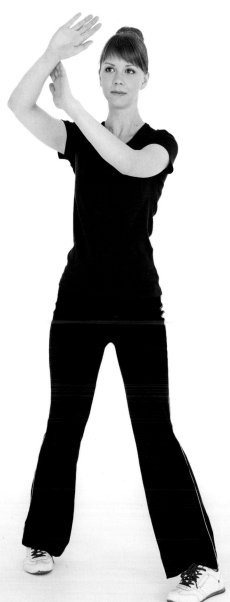

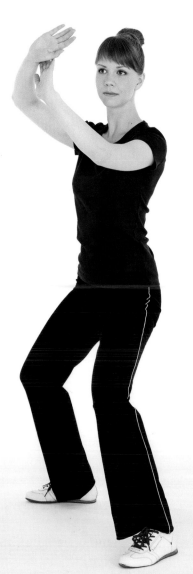

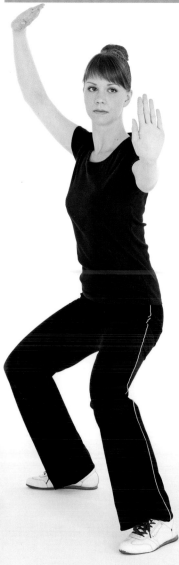

1. Following on from the previous technique, turn the front foot in slightly. Raise and cross the arms.

2. Turn the right foot in the same direction and step back slightly.

3. Open out the arms; extend the left arm forward in a palm strike and raise the right arm above the head. Sink into a horse-riding stance at the same time.

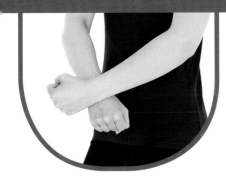

23 Swing Fist

Top tip
• This technique should be performed with a continuous wave-like motion.

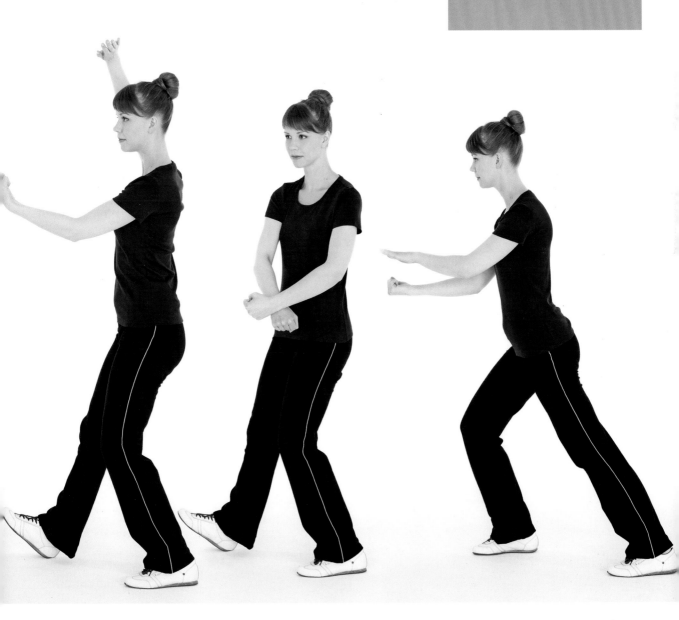

1. Following on from the previous technique, turn the front foot in on the heel and sit back, raising the right arm above the head and uppercutting with the left fist.

2. Turn the body slightly to the left, crossing the arms on the left side, fists clenched.

3. Swing the arms in an arc, strike with the back of the right fist, the left palm on top of the fist and with the weight forward.

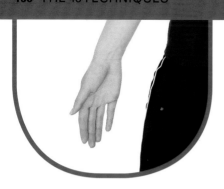

24 Cloud Hands

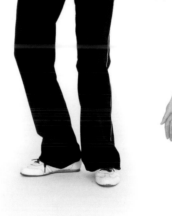

> ## Top tip
> • The circles drawn by the arms are large and the arms should only be slightly bent as they twist and turn.

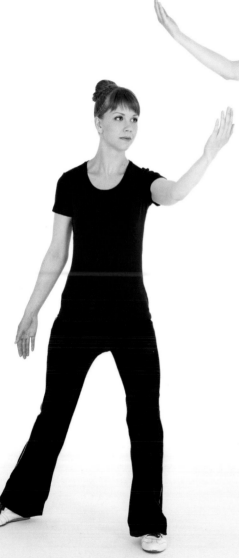

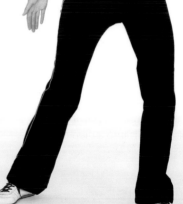

1. Standing with feet a shoulder's width apart, turn, reaching to the left.

2. Draw intersecting clockwise circles in the air.

3. Simultaneously shift the weight and step.

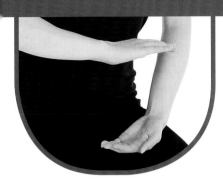

25 Pat the Horse High

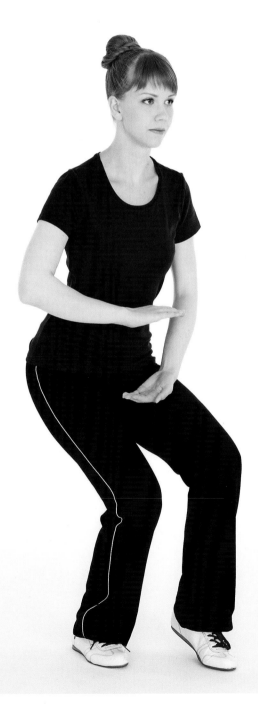

1. Following on from the previous technique, turn left into a high cat stance, left foot forward. The left hand is low and right hand is high, palms facing one another. Sink, bringing the hands in close together.

Top tip

• Contract the torso as you bring the hands in.

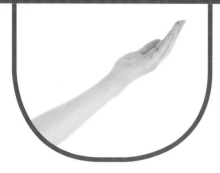

26 Separate Hands

There is only a name for this technique in Wu style, although the posture does exist in other styles.

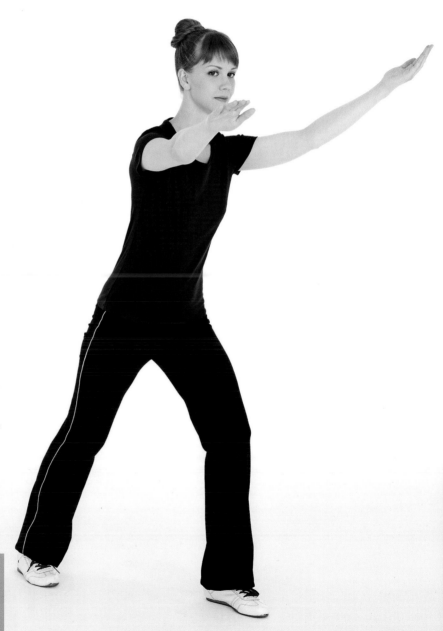

1. Extend the arms out front, with the hand palm up at head level, and the reverse hand palm down and slightly lower, then step into a front stance. The angle between the arms is about 90 degrees and the focus is on the chopping reverse hand.

Top tip

• Get the focus correct; many people stare straight ahead instead of focusing on the striking hand.

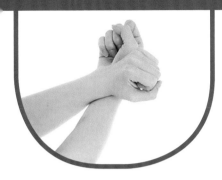

27 Tiger Embraces Head

Another Inner Form technique, Tiger Embraces Head can be practised in a horse-riding stance, twisting the body and limbs from side to side (see page 91).

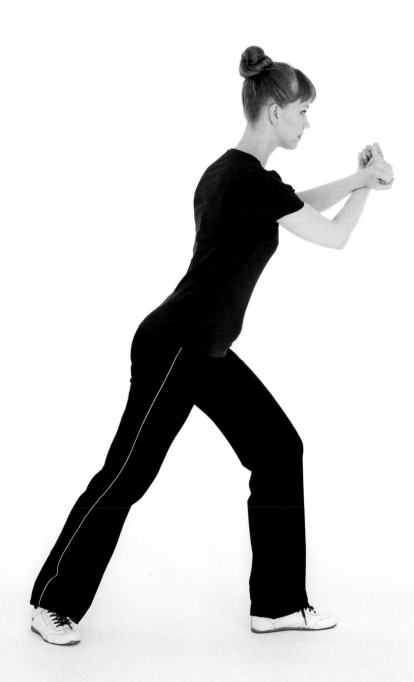

1. Turn the front foot out slightly and, turning the body, clench the fists and cross the arms.

Top tip
• Cross the insides of the wrists when making the crossed arm position.

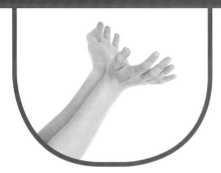

28 Drape Body

Top tip
• The arms and legs are in motion at all times.

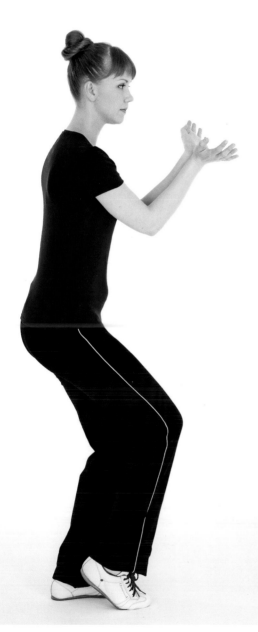

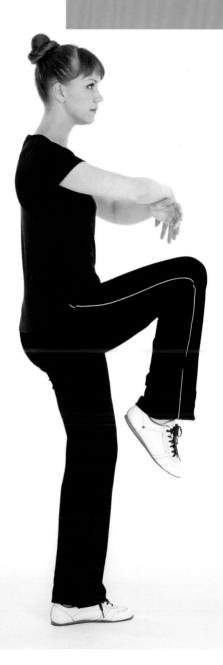

1. Keep the arms together and open the hands.

2. Rotate the arms clockwise and fold them into the chest while raising the right knee.

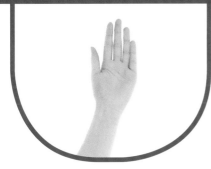

29 Separate Feet

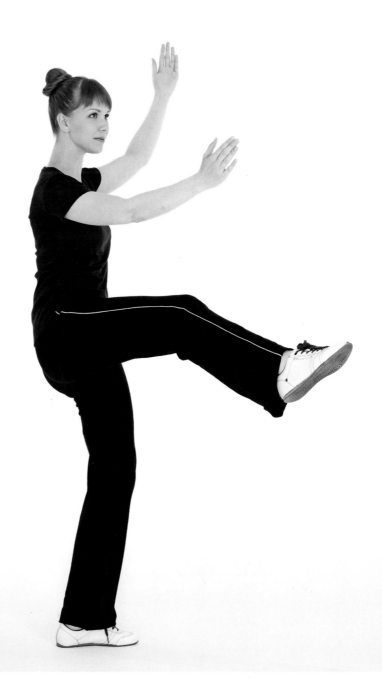

1. Following on from the previous technique, as the arms are crossed, bring the right foot in towards the left foot in a half circle and kick out with the ball of the right foot at 45 degrees, extending the arms. The nose, right foot and arm should all point in the same direction. Extend the left arm back behind the head.

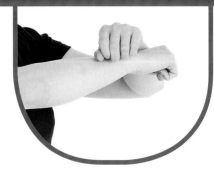

30 Turn Body Kick with Heel

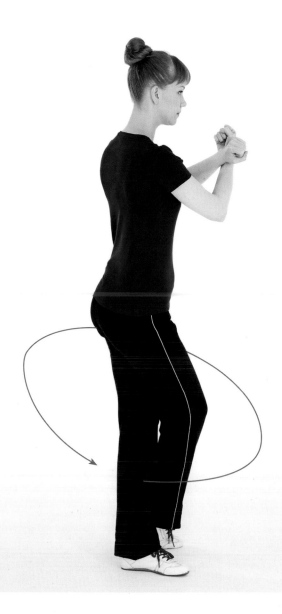

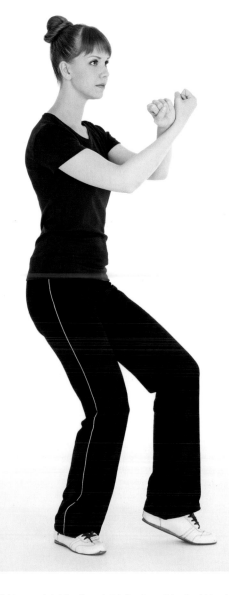

1. Following on from the previous technique, retract the right leg and arm, and cross them over the left leg and arm. Spin on the right heel and ball of the left foot through 315 degrees.

2. Shift the weight to the right foot and ball of the left foot.

Top tip

• The final arm position is the same as in Separate Feet (see page 143).

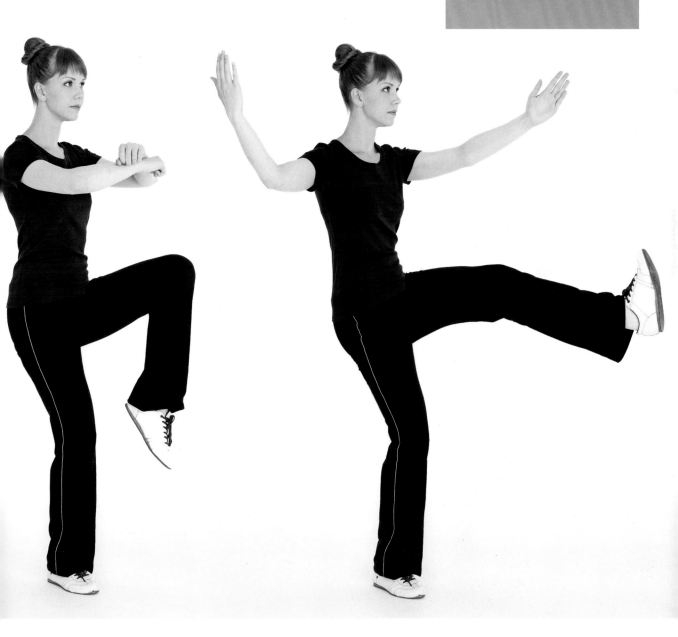

3. Rotate the arms in towards the chest and raise the left knee.

4. Kick out straight ahead with the left heel and extend the arms.

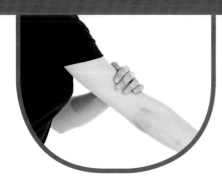

31 Step Forward Plant the Punch

Top tip
• Keep the back straight as you incline forward.

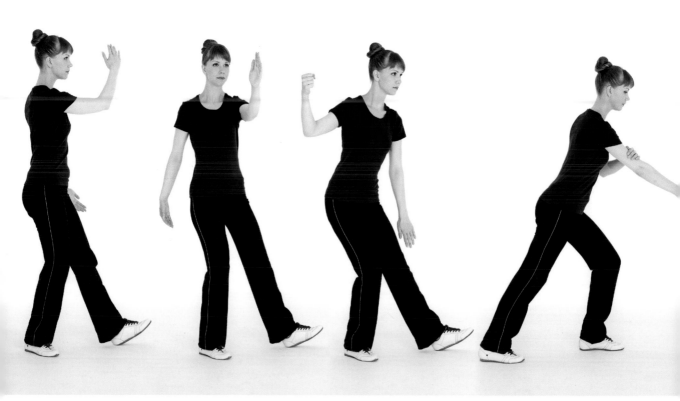

1. Put the left foot forward and down on the heel. Turn the body, and bring the right hand across high.

2. Turn the body to the right and bring the left hand across high.

3. Draw a clockwise circle with the right arm.

4. Shift the weight forward as you punch down through the circle with the right hand.

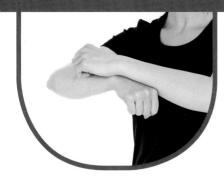

32 Turn Body Swing Fist

Top tip
• This technique comes from high to low, like a wave smashing down.

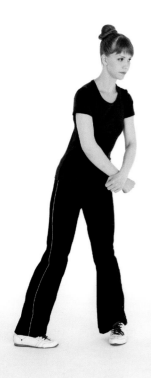 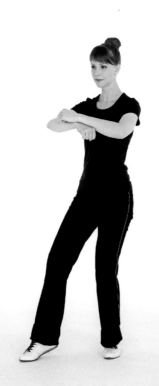 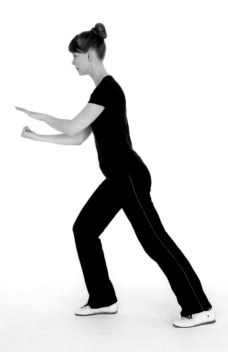

1. Following on from the previous technique, fold the arms and turn the front foot in.

2. Turn around.

3. Step across with the back foot into a front stance, swinging the arms into a backfist and palm strike.

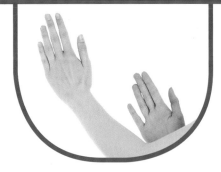

33 Step Back Seven Stars

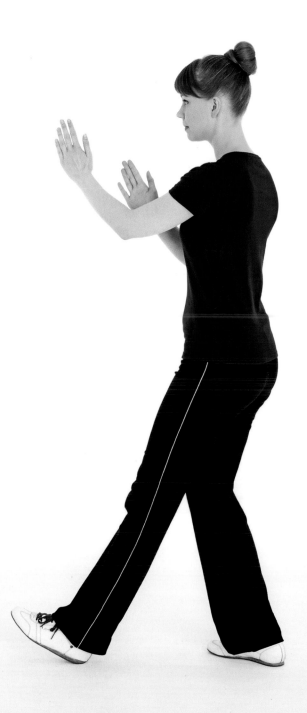

1. Step back diagonally into a Seven Star arm position in a back stance.

Top tip

• Make sure that the front foot and the fingers are all pointing in the same direction.

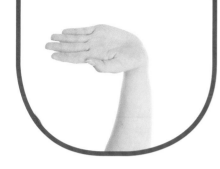

34 Beat the Tiger

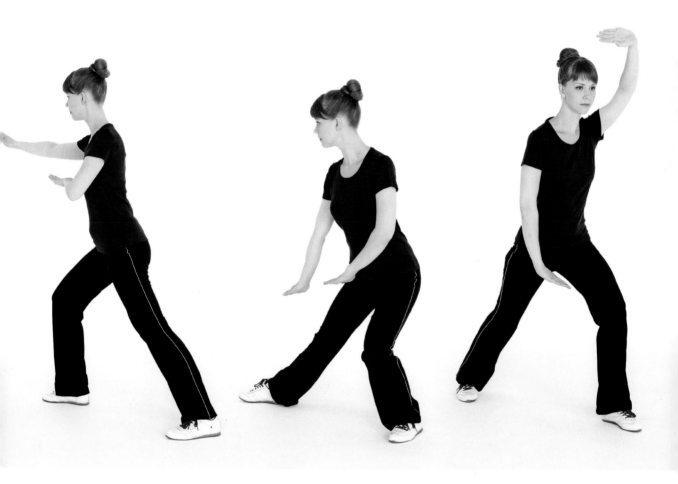

1. Step back into a front stance, with the right hand reaching over the left.

2. Turn the rear foot out while pulling down.

3. Turn round through 180 degrees into a front stance, front hand pushing up, the other hand pushing down; you can have open hands or fists. This is good for stretching the whole body.

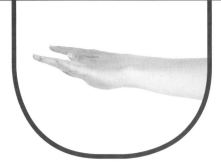

35 Drape Body and Kick

This is also known as Two Raisings of the Foot.

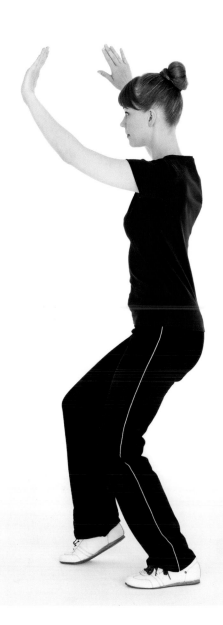

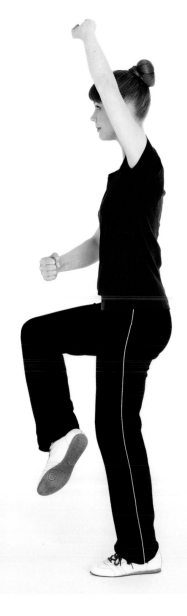

1. Turning the front foot in and pivoting on the rear foot, swing the arms around in a big arc to the right side, sinking as you lower them.

2. Raise the front foot and clench both fists, bringing them into line above the right foot. This line is parallel to the centre line.

Top tip
• Do the turn, pivot and arm swing in one continuous motion.

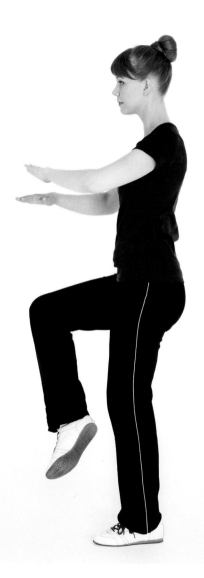

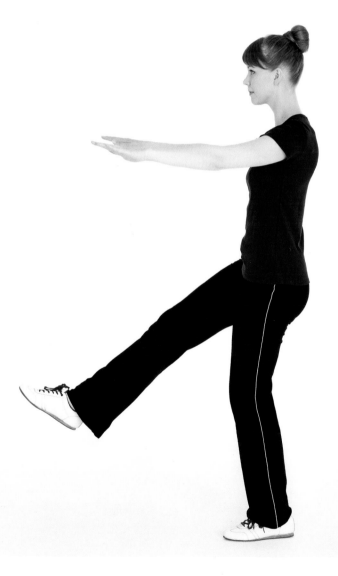

3. Cross the arms in front of the chest.

4. Open and extend the arms at shoulder level; at the same time kick out at knee height.

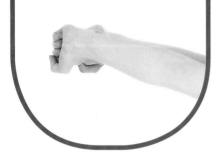

36 Box the Ears

Top tip
• The weight goes forward with the double punch.

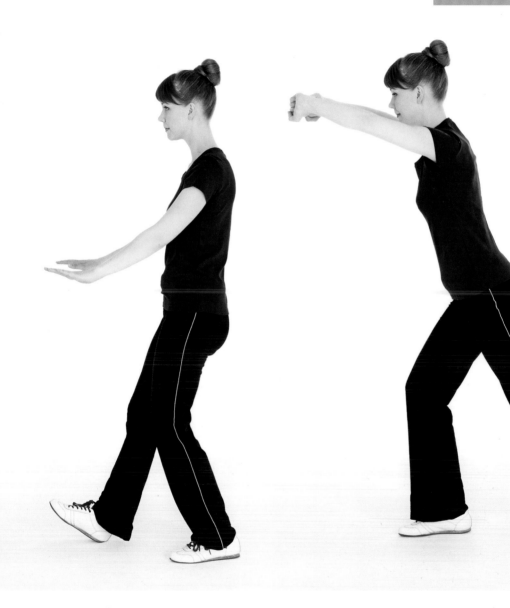

1. Following on from the previous technique, lower the foot and move into a front stance. Bring both arms down to either side in an arc.

2. Lean forward and finish in a double punch at head level.

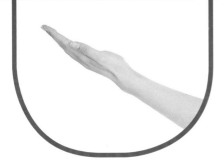

37 Parting Wild Horse's Mane

Top tip
- Get the focus right and show you mean business.

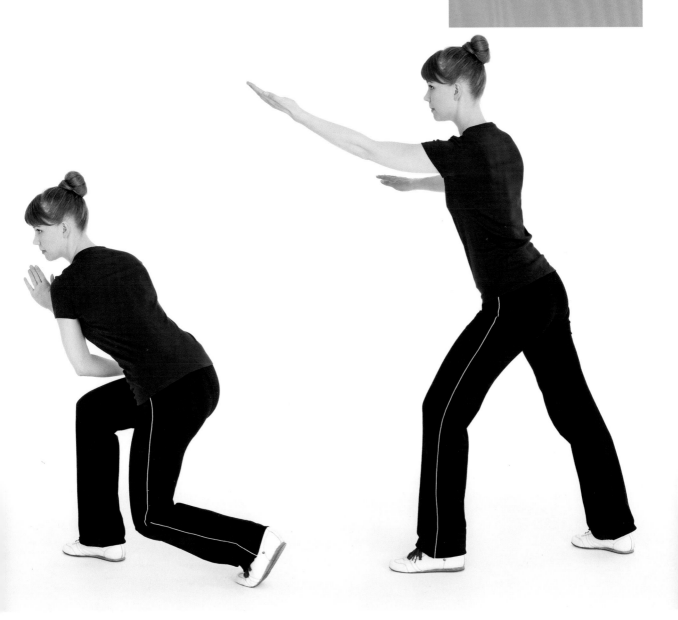

1. Following on from the previous technique, turn the front foot out, twist the body, front hand at face level, other hand low to the side.

2. Step forward into a front stance, opening the arms out at approximately a right angle, front hand palm up, other hand palm down; the focus is on the front hand (note this position is similar to Separate Hands, but the focus is different).

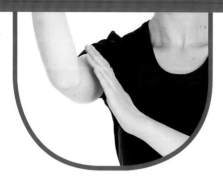

38 Fair Lady Works Shuttle

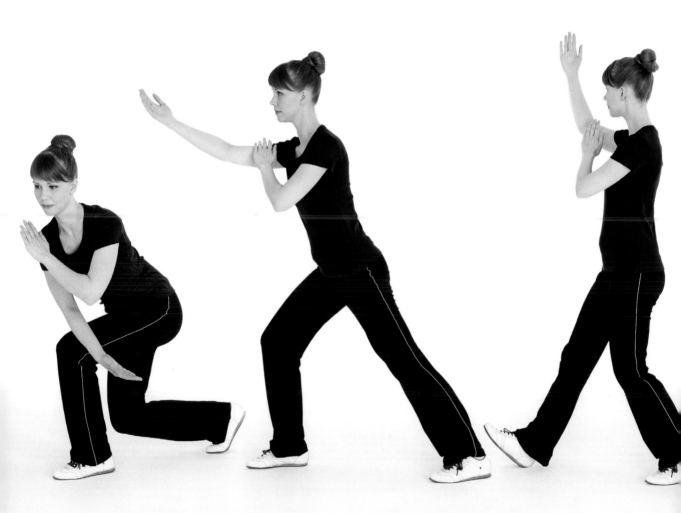

1. Following on from the previous technique, turn the front foot out, twist the body, front hand at face level, other hand low to the side.

2. Step forward into a front stance.

3. Come back on to the heel, swinging the front arm up and to the side.

Top tip
• At the end of the technique, the arms should frame the head.

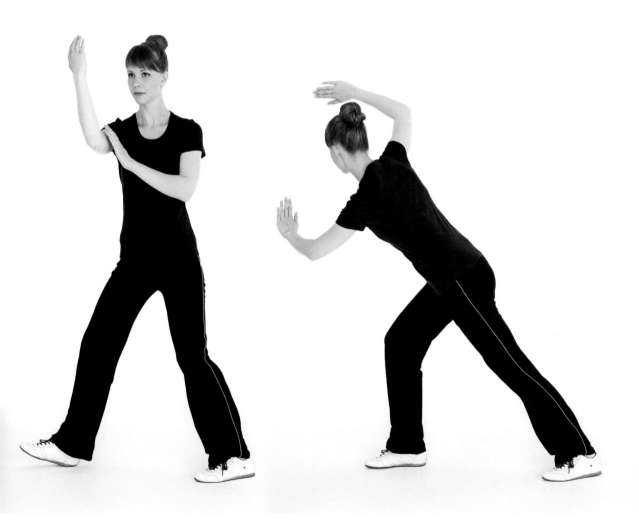

4. Turn to the other side and bring the arms into the chest.

5. Turn back into a front stance, extending the arms with palms out so they face away from the head.

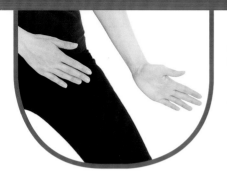

39 Snake Creeps Down (low style)

Top tip
• When you reach over three times, turn the body each time.

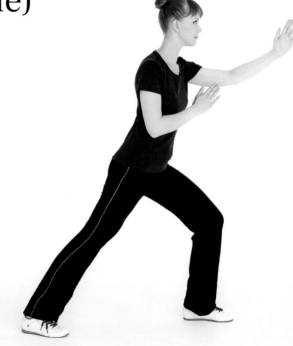

1. Step forward, turn the back foot out and reach over with the left hand, other hand pulled in at the chest.

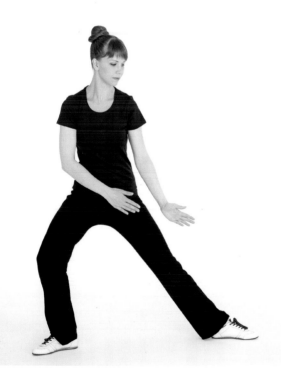

4. Lower the hands, moving into a back stance.

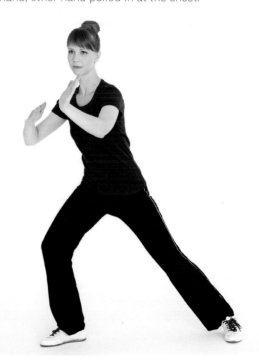

5. Twist the body to bring the hands back, around, up and down in a big circle.

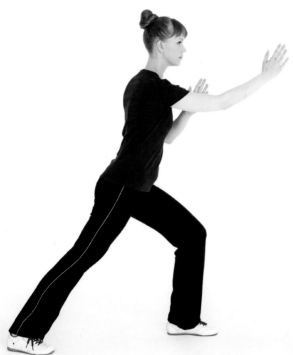

2. Reach over with the right hand.

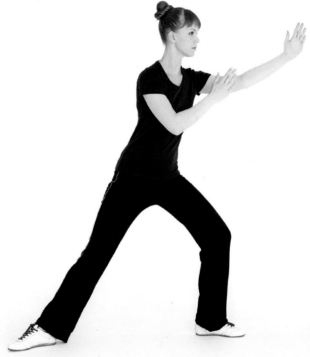

3. Reach with the left hand again, turning the back foot out.

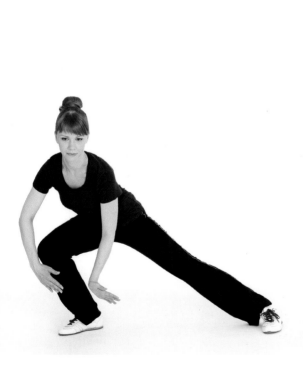

6. When the hands are down, they should be at ankle height.

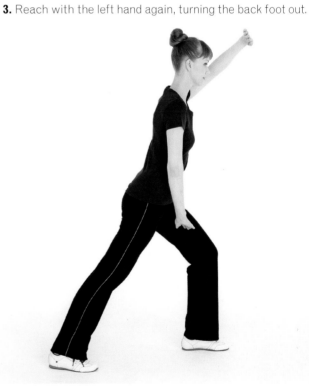

7. Step into a front stance, hands in line, left hand high and right hand low.

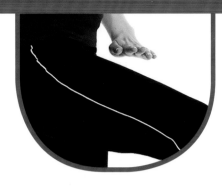

40 Golden Cockerel Stands on One Leg

This technique trains the balance and gives the body a stretch; it can be done slowly and repeatedly on either side to improve blood circulation.

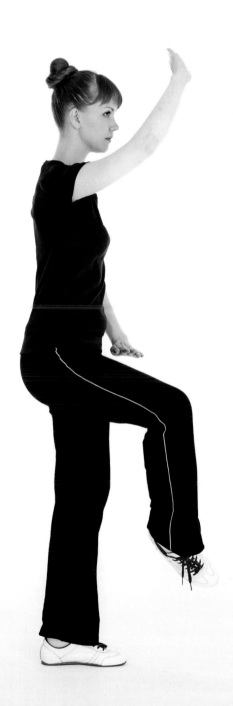

1. Following on from the previous technique, lower the left palm to groin level and raise the right palm above the head. Raise the right foot with the sole turned in. Both hands and the right foot should be in a straight line and parallel to the spine.

Top tip
• Focus on getting the correct alignment.

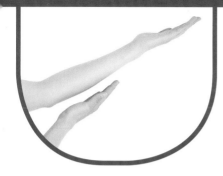

41 White Snake Spits Out Tongue

Top tip
• Make sure that the kick and finger thrust are well-extended as you are in pursuit of a retreating opponent.

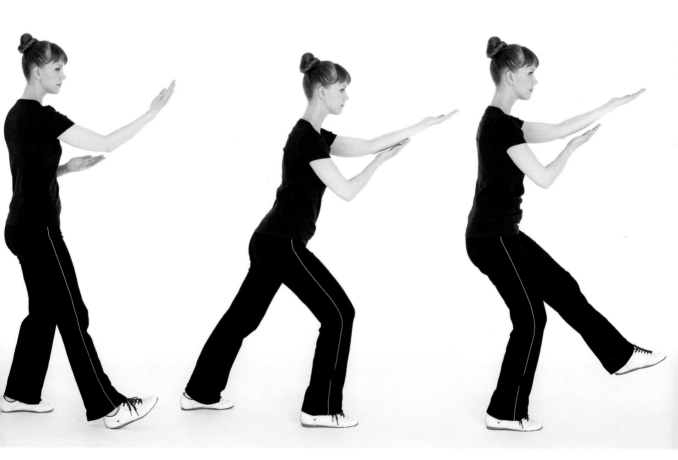

1. Following on from the previous technique, lower the foot into a back stance, bringing the hands in front of the body, right over left and palms up.

2. Shift forward into a front stance, thrusting with the fingers of the left hand.

3. Kick with the left foot.

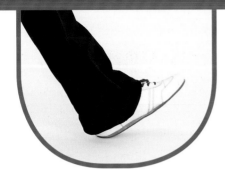

42 Slap the Face

> **Top tip**
> • The heel makes first contact with the ground, then the weight transfers on to the sole.

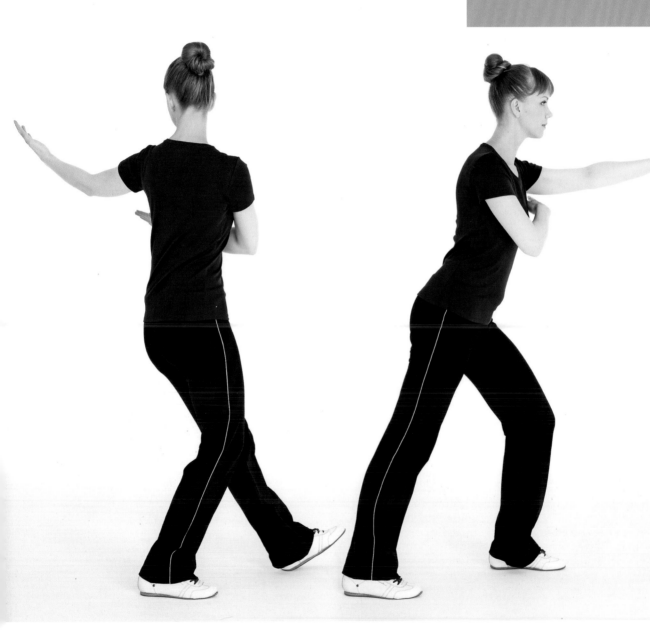

1. Following on from the previous technique, bring the hands around to the left side.

2. Step down into a front stance, slapping forward with the left hand; the right hand protecting the armpit.

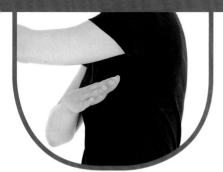

43 Single Hand Sweeps Lotus Leg

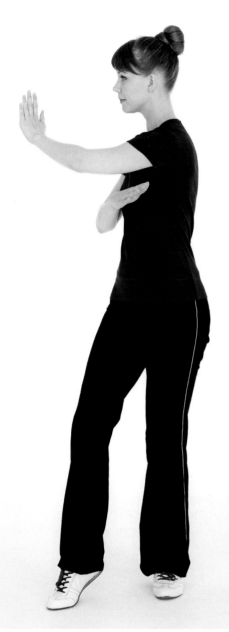

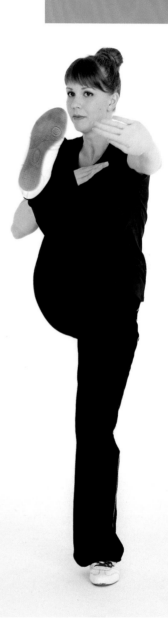

1. Turn the left foot in and pivot on the other foot, turning the body and swinging the left arm around to the right at shoulder level.

2. Raise the right leg and slap the foot with the left hand.

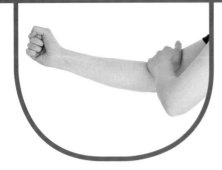

44 Punch the Groin

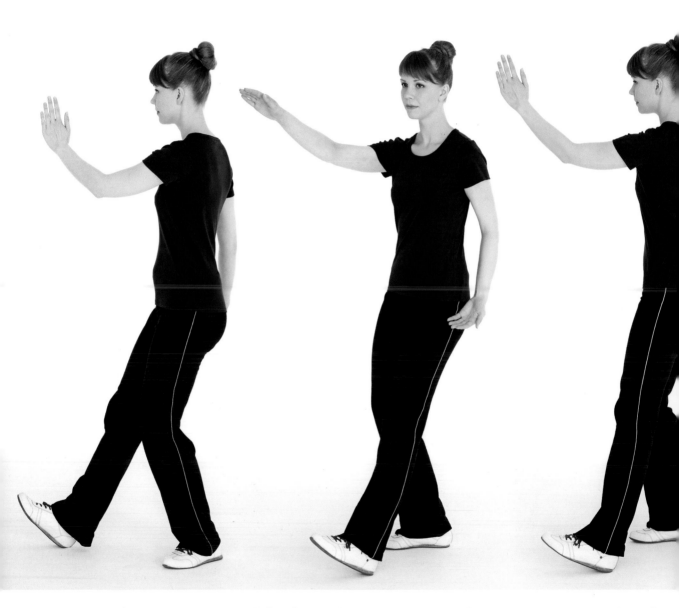

1. Following on from the previous technique; lower the foot.

2. Step forward. Draw clockwise circles with the hands.

3. Draw a clockwise circle in front of the body with the left hand.

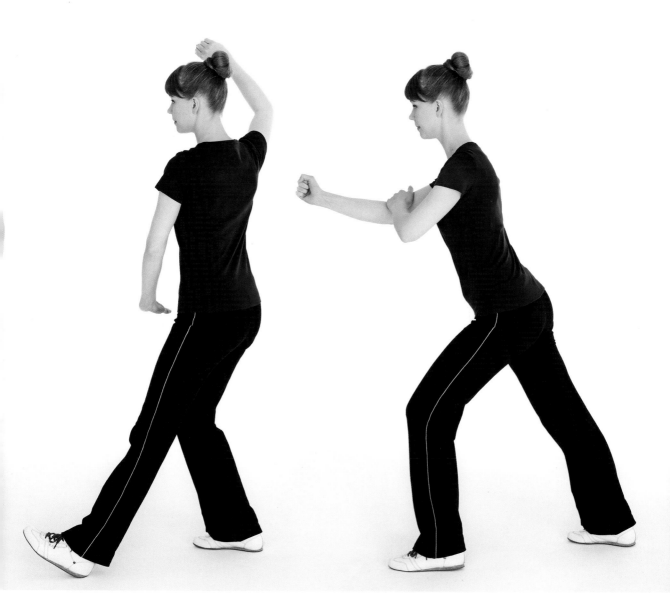

4. At the same time the right fist draws a clockwise circle on the right side.

5. Shift the weight foward. The arms end with an upward punch through the first circle.

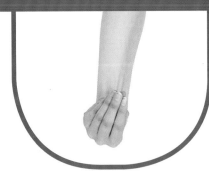

45 Step Back to Ride the Tiger

The details of this technique in *The Classic of Boxing* seem to involve a lot of leg sweeps which are not present in the Tai Chi version.

Top tip
- Sink as the hands go down, rise as they come up.

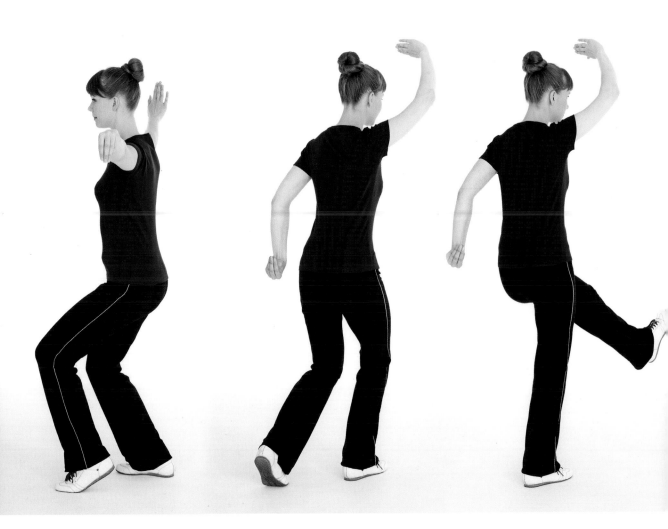

1. Following on from the previous technique, withdraw the front foot a little into a cat stance. Separate the arms and bring them out to the side, right hand palm open, left hand forming a hook.

2. Pivot to the right, scooping down with left hand and raising the right hand above the head.

3. Kick across with the left leg.

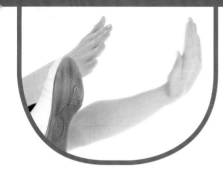

46 Double Hand Sweeps Lotus Leg

Top tip
• Slap the foot with both hands to complete this technique.

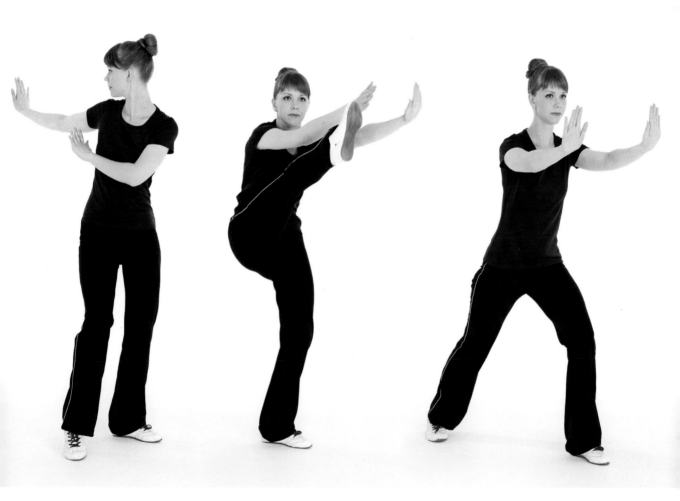

1. Following on from the previous technique, lower the foot, turn it in and pivot on the other foot as you turn, bring the arms round to the right at shoulder level. Turning the centre line, you can see the hands with your peripheral vision.

2. Raise the right leg and slap the foot with both hands.

3. Step back diagonally and push out with both hands.

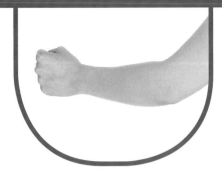

47 Draw the Bow to Shoot the Tiger

Top tip
• Make sure that both fists are punching in the same direction.

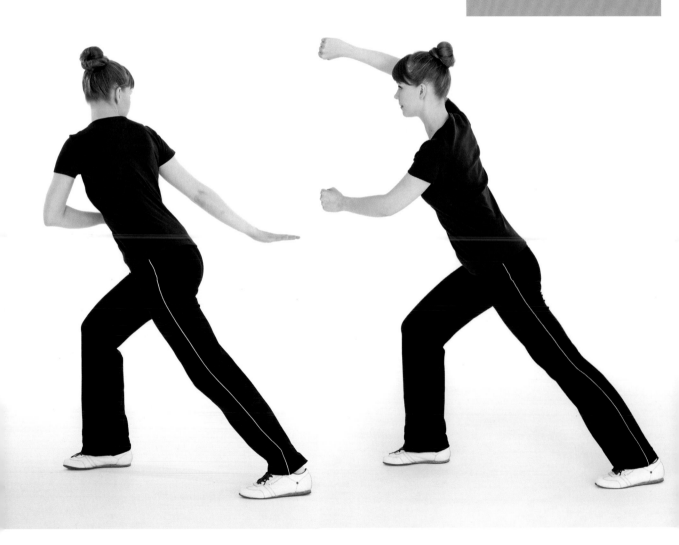

1. Following on from the previous technique, turn the back foot out, lower the hands and swing them round, back, and then to the right as you turn the body.

2. Finish with a double punch.

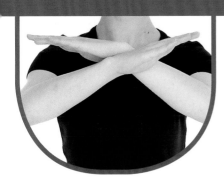

48 Tai Chi in Unity

Top tip
• The focus follows the finger thrust.

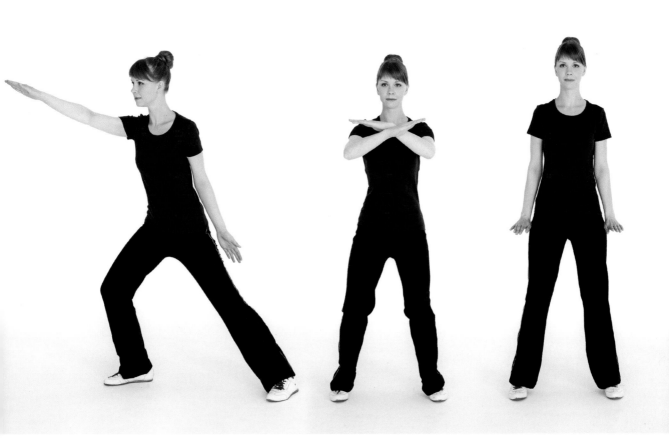

1. Following on from the previous technique, turn the front foot in slightly and thrust diagonally forward with the fingers of the right hand as the left hand comes back low.

2. Step up with the back foot so the feet are a shoulder's width apart, bring the hands into the chest, left over right. Bend the knees.

3. Tai Chi at Rest – back where we started (see page 112).

8 Tai Chi in Application

'To see what is righteous and not act is to be without courage.'

It seems pointless to claim that you practise Tai Chi as a martial art and yet be unable to use your skills when it is appropriate to do so.

One Saturday night many years ago, I put on my best suit and tie and went with my brother Steve to the Horseshoe Bar in Glasgow, where both my granddads used to drink, to attend the stag night of our brother James. Hours later, when the pub closed, Steve and I went to Central Station to join the long queue for taxis. After a bit, a rough-looking fellow came up and in an assured way put his arm round the girl queuing behind me, just as a boyfriend would do. He became more familiar, pulling her head close so he could whisper something to her. She appeared distressed. People started to stare. I watched what was happening, but said nothing. He barged me from behind. I withstood it. He made a rude and untrue sexual insinuation. Knife attacks are common in Glasgow, so I turned and punched him. I followed up with a couple of kicks to bring him to his knees. I advised the fellow in Glasgow patois to desist and depart. He limped off into the night. The girl said, 'Thanks, mister, I didn't know him at all.' Everybody stared. Three of Glasgow's boys in blue walked past. Steve and I got into a taxi. Steve said, 'I was thinking of doing something…'

I learned something from the experience. I've stopped joining taxi queues – I now take the bus.

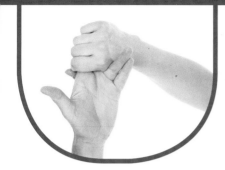

Shuai Jiao, Die Pu, Qin Na

Many Tai Chi practitioners have heard of San Shou/Scattering Hands, which can refer to free fighting or to the self-defence applications of a specific martial art. If you want to claim you practise Chinese martial arts, you should also understand the terms Shuai Jiao, Die Pu and Qin Na.

All three of these skills are part of the repertoire of San Shou techniques used in Tai Chi Chuan and other Chinese martial arts; they are not separate arts in themselves, but are a useful way to group and analyse techniques. This is rather complex because many Tai Chi techniques have multiple applications and can be combined with others to make even more. Thus, one technique with its different applications could legitimately be classified as belonging to all three of Shuai Jiao, Die Pu and Qin Na.

In recent years Shuai Jiao has become a reasonably well-known term through the tournaments held in the Far East, Europe and North America. It is not necessary to wear the special tournament pyjamas in order to practise the art and such tournaments are as representative of Shuai Jiao as Judo tournaments are of Jujutsu or as Pushing Hands tournaments are of Tai Chi. Likewise, a lot of people think of Qin Na purely in terms of joint locks and while this is certainly part of what Qin Na can be, there is a bit more to it.

Many Chinese characters like Shuai are composed of a radical which gives a clue as to the meaning, and a phonetic which gives the sound. The radical for the character Shuai is the character for hand, while the phonetic represents a net with a frame, such as is used to snare birds, and a rope which is used to make the trap fall.

Shuai thus means to throw to the ground or to shake. Jiao is nowadays usually given as either the character meaning mutually – so mutually throwing to the ground is wrestling – or the character meaning the bones of the leg, suggesting the use of tripping and sweeping in wrestling. Another variation is the Jiao character meaning horn(s).

Other terms used to refer to wrestling include Jiao Di and Jiao Li. Here the Jiao character means horns, while Di means to resist and Li is strength. It is believed that contestants originally put on horned headgear and tried to butt and gore one another; of course, even without such headgear, butting could be a useful tactic.

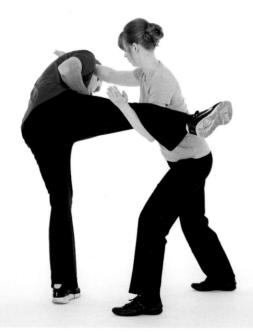

1. Trap the kicking leg.

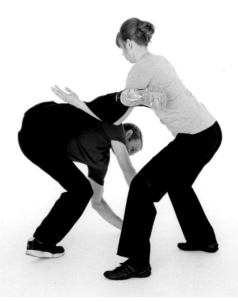

2. Shuai jiao: a grappling takedown against a roundhouse kick.

During the Tang dynasty, the term Xiang Pu referred to wrestling contests. Xiang means mutually, while Pu is striking/leaning against/falling. This same Pu character is used in the Tai Chi technique Pu Mian Zhang, literally strike face palm or, more colloquially, Slap the Face.

The term Die Pu is almost unknown. In 2001 I attended a lecture in Paris given by a Czech academic and Chen stylist who spoke fluent Chinese; he'd never heard of it. Die means fall/stumble while Pu again is striking/leaning against/falling. This suggests a little more than simple wrestling. In Tai Chi there are two parts to Die Pu. First we try to evade and/or to redirect the opponent's attack and then to counterattack, throwing him to the ground and setting up the possibility of a follow-up strike or lock, as shown in the form technique Plant the Punch. Another way is to reverse this as in Flying Oblique, whereby, if we are being held, we can use a strike or strikes (Pu) to distract the opponent and force him to release his grip or hold, enabling us to counter him with a throw (Die). In the main, Die Pu is a counter-attacking method.

Qin Na means seizing and holding. Usually we are trying to seize and hold the joints, since these are also nerve centres and can be struck or used as levers to manipulate the opponent's body, but such seizing can also be applied to the torso, hair, genitalia and clothes. The holding aspect can either be to control the opponent prior to using pressure points on him, or simply to restrain him as a police officer or security guard might. I used this skill a number of times when making arrests, particularly when commanding the Kowloon Regional Vice Squad.

Putting It into Practice

Having understood the theory, we come to the method of practice. In Tai Chi, we can practise San Shou techniques in a variety of ways. Hand Form practice is important, as in many instances movements which occur in the Hand Form either set up the next technique or are applied if the preceding technique has been resisted. However, partnered practice is more important, taking turns to apply the technique on an attacker, or as part of an arsenal of techniques to be used in freestyle practice. Many Die Pu and most Qin Na techniques can also be practised as part of Pushing Hand drills such as Four Corners, Four Directions, Zhou Lu and so on, or as part of freestyle Moving Step Pushing Hands.

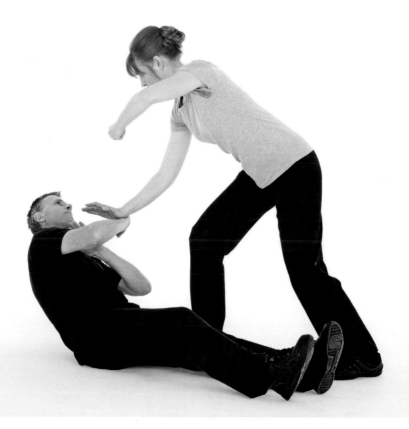

Die pu: a counter-attacking method. Make your opponent fall, then strike.

Many Tai Chi terms are poorly understood and badly explained. For example, one of the old names for Tai Chi Chuan, the 13 Postures or Tactics, should not be defined as narrowly as it is in many styles. These tactics are only a rough guide and are not as distinct as many would like to believe. For example, Pat The Horse High can be applied with elements of An and Lie and Looking Left or Right, while Single Hand Seize Leg can contain elements of Peng and Cai along with Advance or Step Back. These are quite different explanations of these tactics to those given in most books, which completely fail to explain such applications.

The main reason that most masters, whether Chinese or Western, have such conservative and limited views on these 13 Tactics is that their knowledge of San Shou is also limited. They are like the frog at the bottom of the well in the Chinese proverb, believing that the small stretch of sky overhead is all there is. Techniques and tactics have to be multi-dimensional or what is being practised is not a martial art, but some kind of museum piece.

Some Confusion with Names

Many techniques have, through problems of incorrect transcription or different dialects, lost their original names and ended up with similar-sounding or similarly written names – for example what in most Tai Chi styles is known as Shan Tong Bei/Fan Through the Back is in Wu Yuxiang known as San Tong Bei/Three Changes of the Back.

In other cases techniques have been entirely renamed or have come to have more than one name. For example Tai Chi's famous advanced Pushing Hands exercise, widely known as Da Lu, has two other names, both of which are much more expressive of the purpose of the exercise than Da Lu, which merely means Big Diversion to the Side – hardly poetic.

In yet other cases, names have been lost because the technique was kept secret or due to negligence. One of the 40 writings presented by Yang Banhou to the Wu family (I've referred to these writings elsewhere in this book) gives a whole list of technique names, all of which have been lost or have fallen out of use.

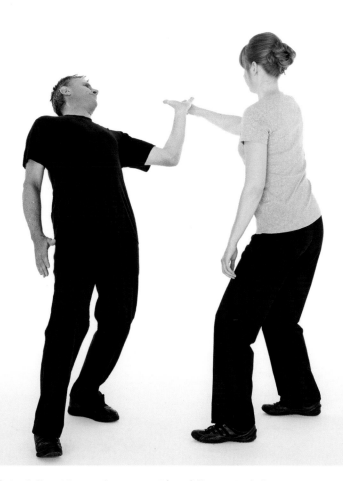

Qin Na: seizing and holding. Potentially setting up the opponent for a follow-up technique.

Fundamental Applications

Certain Tai Chi techniques can be considered fundamental in that they can be found in almost all styles. We are now going to look at the application of some of these fundamental techniques.

For comparison purposes, each fundamental application includes line drawings of each technique as it appears in the Long Forms of the five famous Tai Chi families (see also the 48 Techniques, Chapter 7). All these forms have been simplified over the years, so differences are considerable. This is particularly the case with my version of certain techniques such as Beginning Style which contain Inner Form techniques (Vanguard Arms).

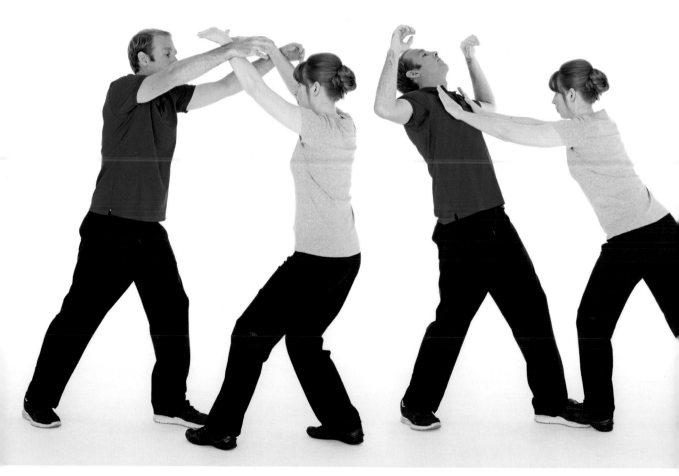

1. Step back arching the wrists in an upward parry, against an attempted strangle, then close the distance with a kick and a push.

2. Close the distance, stamp on his front foot and hit him with a double palm strike.

Beginning Style

Every form has a beginning; every beginning style has a purpose.

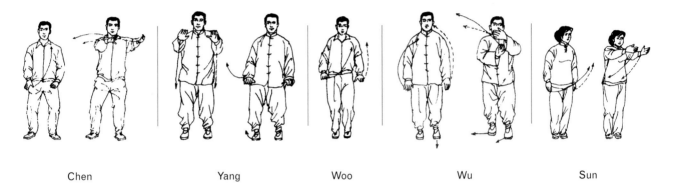

Chen   Yang   Woo   Wu   Sun

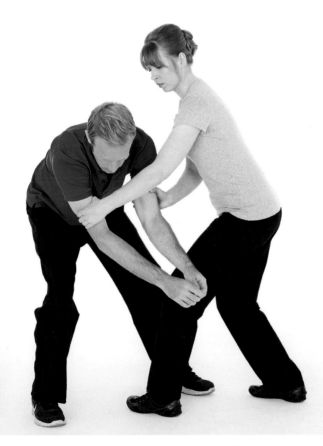

3. An alternative counter is to suddenly sink and jerk the opponent off-balance.

Vanguard Arms

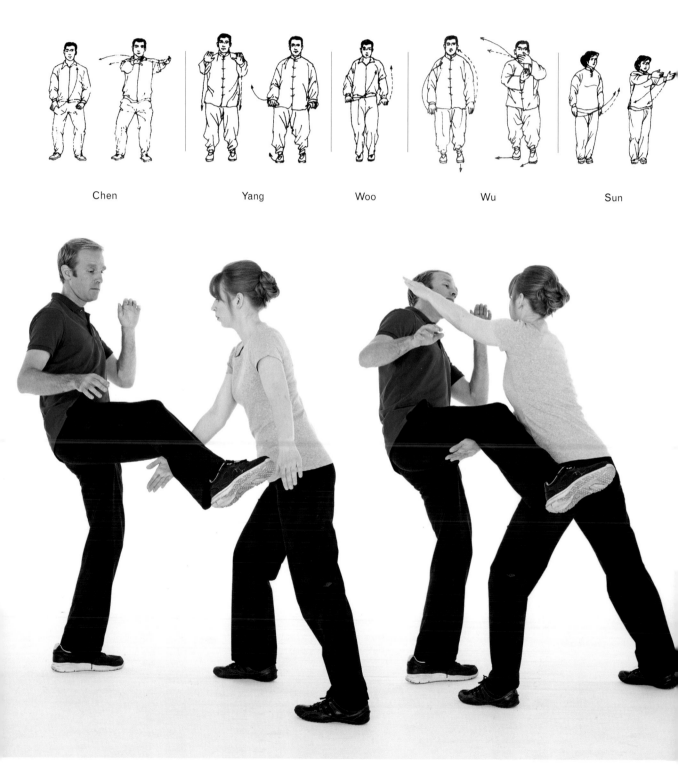

Chen   Yang   Woo   Wu   Sun

1. She evades her opponent and slaps aside his kick.

2. She steps forward and strikes her opponent's head with her left hand.

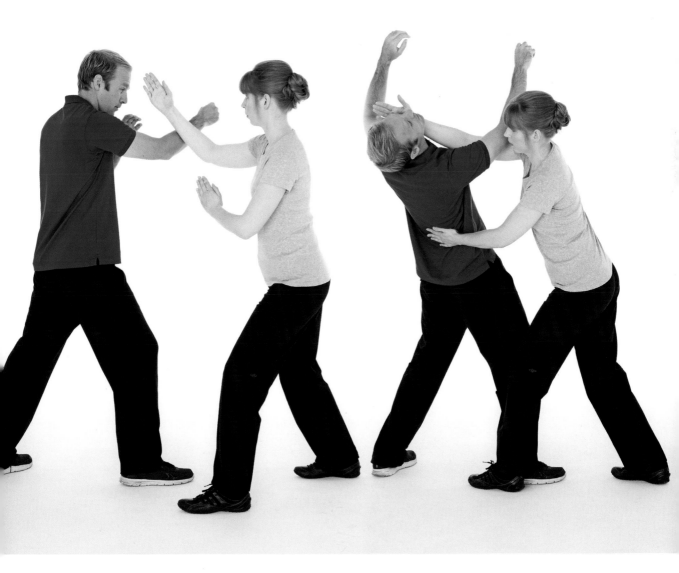

1. She evades her opponent and intercepts his punch.

2. She steps in and simultaneously strikes her opponent in the face and kidney while tripping/sweeping his front foot.

Seven Stars

The Classic of Boxing states that in Seven Star Fists,
'Hands and legs are coordinated.
Step by step press, above and below raise the cage.
Even if he has fast hands and feet like the wind,
I also can disturb and rush him, chopping heavily.'

There are a number of Seven Star techniques in
Tai Chi Chuan – sometimes used as a guard, sometimes
applied with fists, sometimes with open hands. It can
involve chopping, as here. The second sentence just
quoted advises us not to rush.

The cage can be the arms, or a reference to lifting
heavy objects to strengthen the arms, such as carrying
a cage, but more likely it refers to using a guard.
Disturbing the opponent suggests using feints to distract
him before attacking.

In the Long Form we have Seven Stars, Step Back
Seven Stars and Step Up Seven Stars.

Variation 1

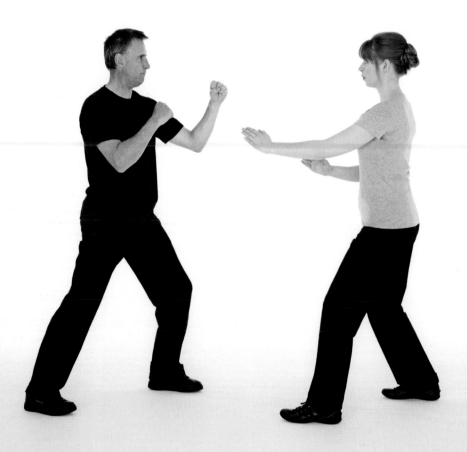

The Seven Star guard.

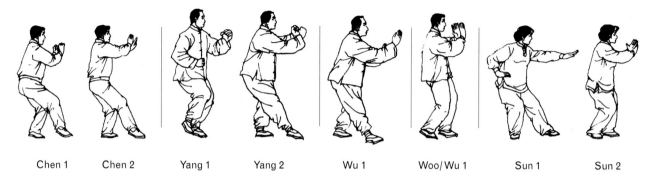

| Chen 1 | Chen 2 | Yang 1 | Yang 2 | Wu 1 | Woo/ Wu 1 | Sun 1 | Sun 2 |

Variation 2

Variation 3

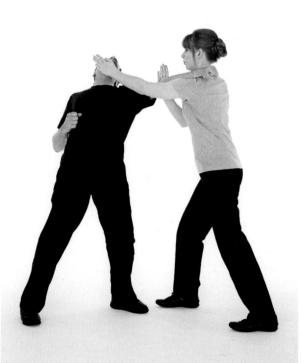

Use the Seven Star step to avoid your opponent's punch, giving a double-impact palm strike to his arm.

Alternatively, combine a soft interception with a horizontal face slap.

Variation 4

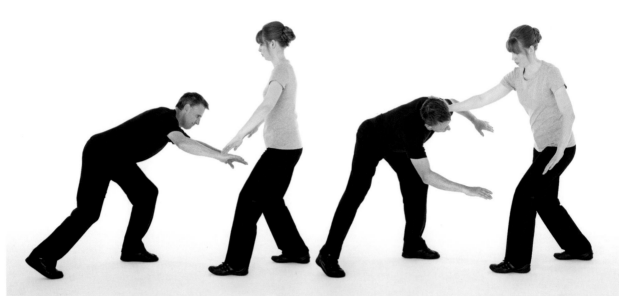

1. If an opponent attempts to grab your arms when they are in the Seven Star guard, collapse the guard. This will make him stagger forward off balance.

2. Step in slightly to counter with a palm strike.

Variation 5

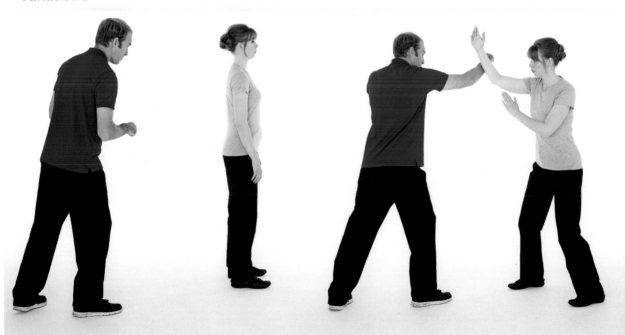

1. Your peripheral vision allows you to notice an assailant behind you and to your right.

2. Turn and raise your right arm to help form Seven Stars, with which you intercept and control your opponent.

Different applications using Seven Stars

The variations demonstrated show that:

- Seven Stars can be a guard (see Variation 1)
- Seven Stars can be a double-impact strike on the opponent's striking arm (see Variation 2).
- Seven Stars can be a diversion and face slap (see Variation 3).
- Seven Stars guard can be used to unbalance an opponent by collapsing it when he tries to attack (see Variation 4).
- Seven Stars can be used to intercept an attack from the side, countering with a finger thrust into soft tissue (see Variation 5).
- Step Back Seven Stars involves uprooting the opponent (see Variation 6).
- In Step Up Seven Stars we catch the opponent's foot and flip him after giving him a low kick (see Variation 7).

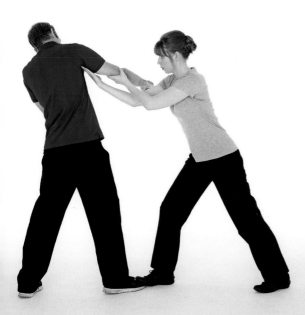

3. Controlling your opponent's arm, give a finger thrust to his armpit.

Top tip
- Keep changing the angle on your opponent.

Variation 6

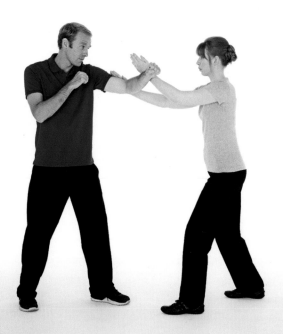 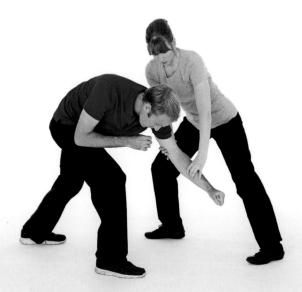

1. Avoid and intercept your attacker's head punch.

2. Step back suddenly and pull down, uprooting and unbalancing him.

Variation 7

Capture the opponent's kick and lift his leg, then follow up with a low kick to the groin or to the supporting leg.

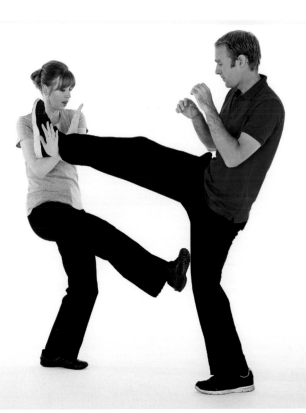

Single Whip

The Classic of Boxing states,
'Bent Single Whip, Yellow Flower advances urgently ['Yellow Flower' is a metaphor for virgin, so step like a virgin with closed legs when you advance].
Open and lift his legs, left and right it is difficult for him to defend.
Snatch step [a lunge step as in fencing] and use the fist continuously to chop the front.
Chen Xiang gesture/style, push over Tai Shan.'

The significance of the last gesture is that Chen Xiang's mother had the mountain of Tai Shan put on top of her and Chen lifted it off.

Single Whip is one of the techniques common to all Tai Chi Chuan styles, though there are considerable variations in execution. In my Wu lineage, the technique is executed in a horse-riding stance when it is performed in Hand Form. It is also one of the most repeated techniques in the Long Form, occurring more than ten times in the one I practise. This gives some hint as to its importance.

When talking of Hand Form Single Whip, many exponents tend to think of the completed position but, at its most sophisticated, there is much coiling and uncoiling of arms, legs and torso before arriving at that point.

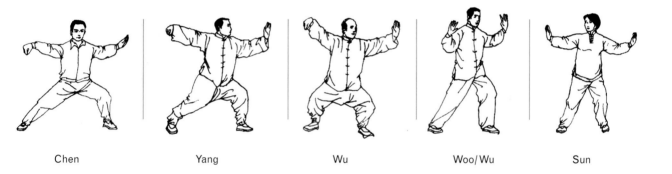

| Chen | Yang | Wu | Woo/Wu | Sun |

Variation 1

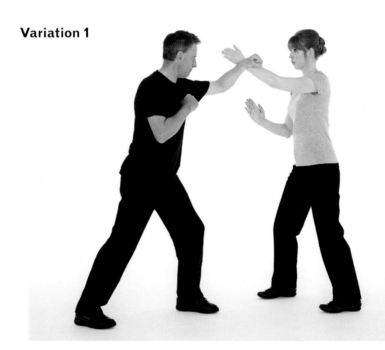

Sidestep and intercept the opponent's attack with a sliding defence.
[Continued overleaf]

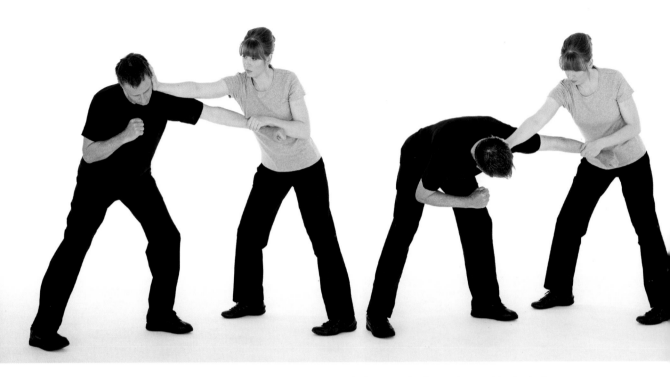

2. Seize his wrist and strike his head.

3. Put your bodyweight into the technique.

Variation 2

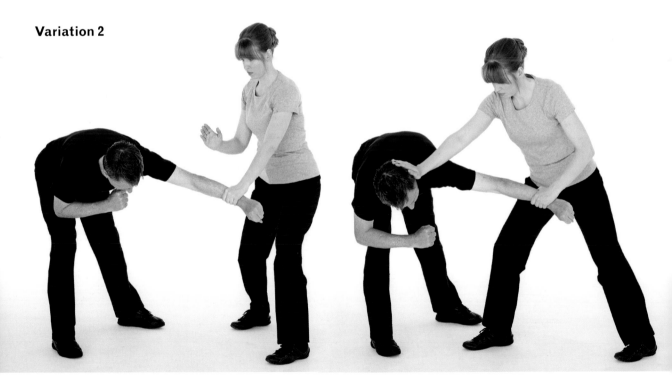

1. After intercepting the attack, seize your opponent's arm and jerk him forward off balance – this also shakes up his nervous system.

2. He is defenceless against the palm strike.

Variation 3

Counter a kick with a knee defence and slap the opponent's face.

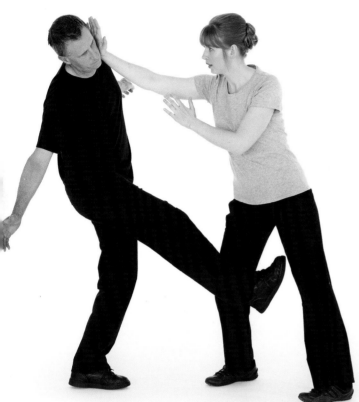

Variation 4

Use a turn of the body and a sliding defence against your opponent's swing; at the same time counter with a swing of your own, striking with the back of the wrist.

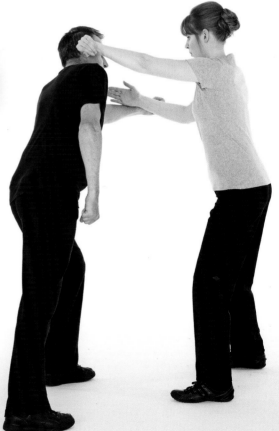

Variation 5

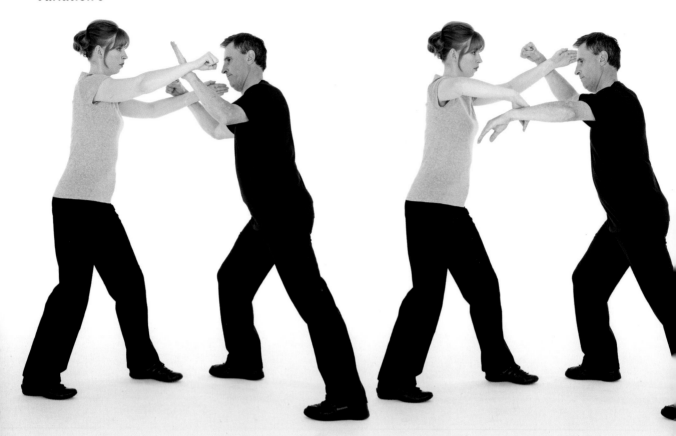

1. Your opponent blocks your swing.

2. Respond by hooking his blocking arm away.

Variation 3, with knee defence to a kick and simultaneous slap, could certainly fit the explanations in the first two sentences of the quotation given on page 181. The hooked strike with the back of the wrist could be interpreted as a chop. 'Pushing over Tai Shan' could refer to the palm strike to the head.

There are suggestions in Chinese martial arts circles that there was also a Double Whip, whether in Tai Chi or otherwise, but it's a known unknown; no-one really knows. There is also the idea that the body is the stock of the whip and the arms the lash. Single Whip exists in external martial arts such as Long Boxing, where it ends in a front stance with fists extended. In Tai Chi applications of Single Whip the fists are not used, so the Long Boxing version is much closer to that described in *The Classic of Boxing*.

The hooked hand is sometimes said to be brandishing a whip as if on horseback (the Wu family descended from Manchu bannermen and were renowned horsemen).

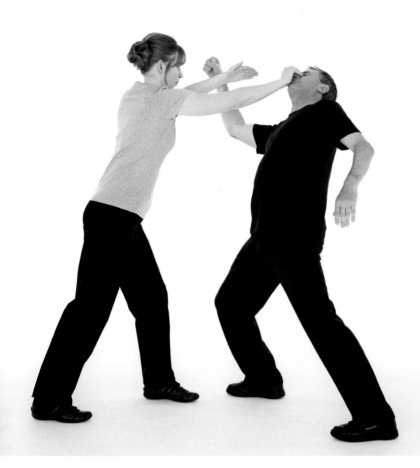

3. Counter with a strike to the eyes, using your fingertips in a sort of pecking position.

Variation 6

Move back slightly, brushing the attack past you and countering with a back-of-the-hand strike of your own.

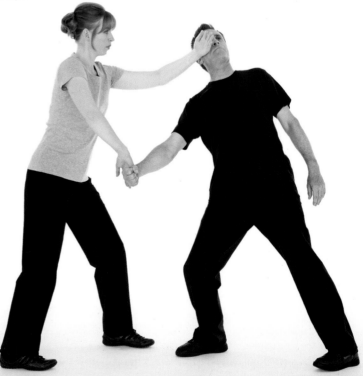

Grasping Bird's Tail

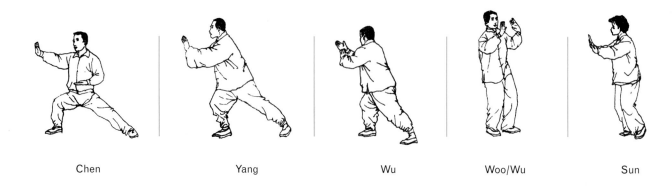

| Chen | Yang | Wu | Woo/Wu | Sun |

Variation 1

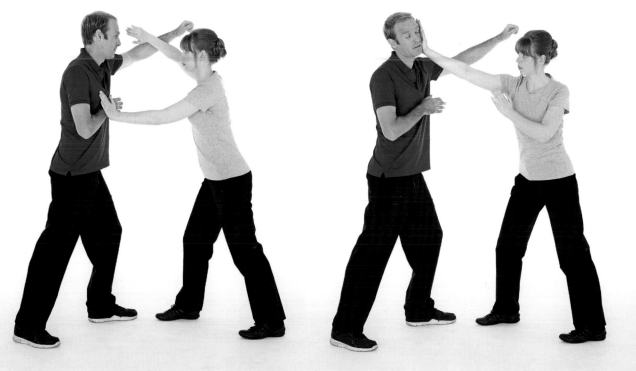

1. Turn and raise your right arm in a sliding defence against a swing to the head, at the same time jamming your opponent's other hand against his body.

2. Strike your attacker immediately with your defending hand.

Variation 2

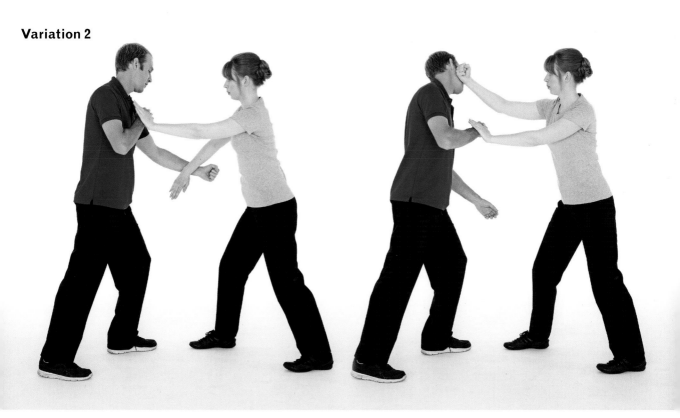

1. Turn and lower your right arm in a sliding defence against his swing to your body, simultaneously jamming his other hand against his body.

2. Strike your attacker immediately with your defending hand.

Variation 3

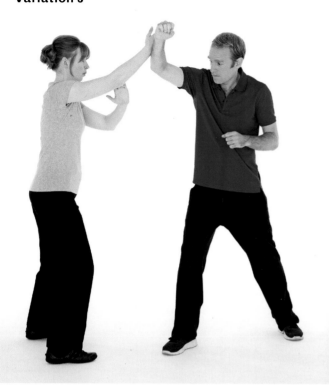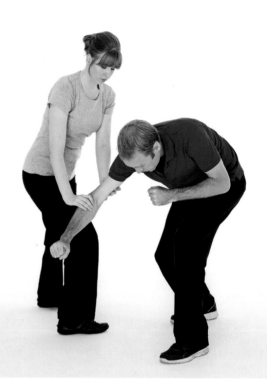

1. Turn and raise your right arm to intercept the attacker's hammer-fist blow to your head.

2. Pull down suddenly to uproot him.

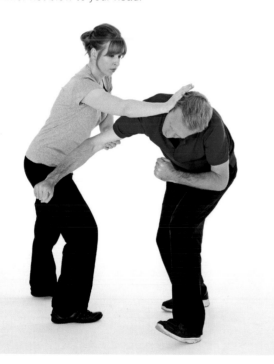

3. Complete the technique with a palm strike.

Tiger Embraces Head

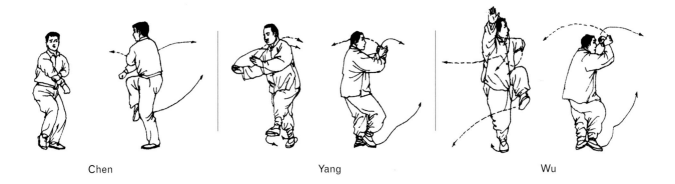

Chen   Yang   Wu

Variation 1

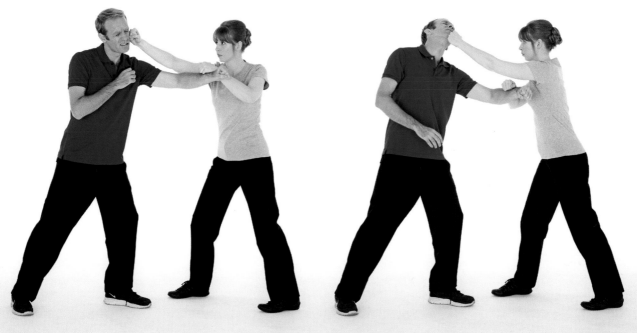

1. Sidestep your opponent's attack, while at the same time intercepting and countering.

2. Make sure with another counter.

Variation 2

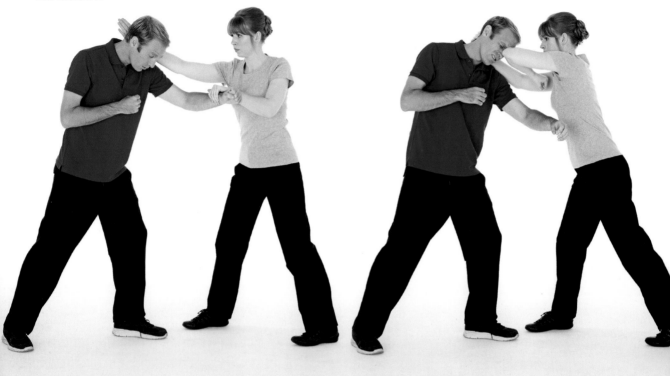

1. Sidestep and intercept your opponent's attack, slapping the back of his head.

2. Follow up by pulling him onto a forearm smash.

Variation 3

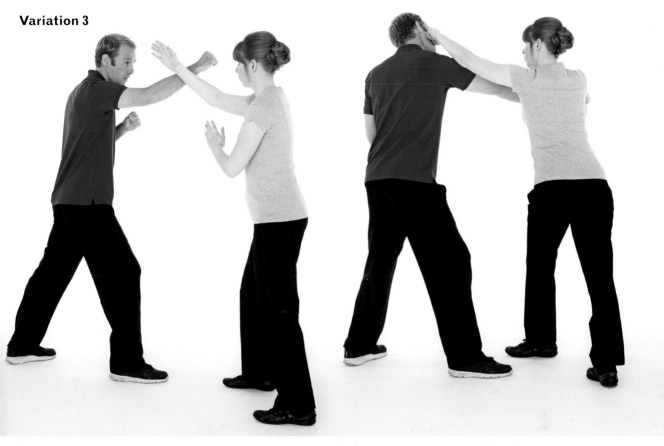

1. Intercept the attack to the head.

2. Step across and inside with a slicing punch.

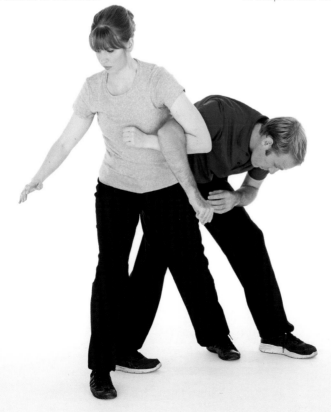

3. Use your opponent's arm as a lever to unbalance him or to use him as a shield.

Golden Cockerel on One Leg

'Golden Cockerel on One
Leg, preparing to rise.
Pull back the leg(s) while
giving a crosswise punch.
Snatch with the Back, Reclining Ox double fall.
After this my opponent incessantly
complains to high heaven.'

Golden Cockerel on One Leg is a classical Tai Chi Chuan
technique. It requires the boxer to be erect and prepared
to fight like a cockerel, maybe with one foot on tiptoe.

Line three of the verse describes the posture in the
illustration, pulling back the right leg.

Line five seems to describe throwing the opponent
over the back; using the bodyweight rather than
the arms makes my attack heavy, as the weight of an
ox and 'double fall' suggests I land on him to give a
double impact. This is unlike any Tai Chi application of
this technique that I have ever seen.

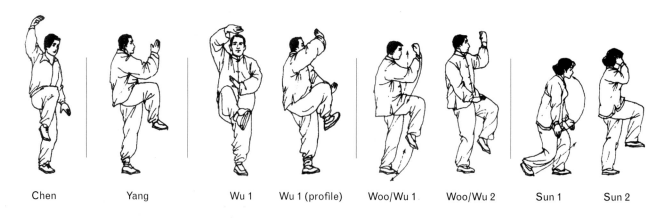

Chen   Yang   Wu 1   Wu 1 (profile)   Woo/Wu 1   Woo/Wu 2   Sun 1   Sun 2

Variation 1

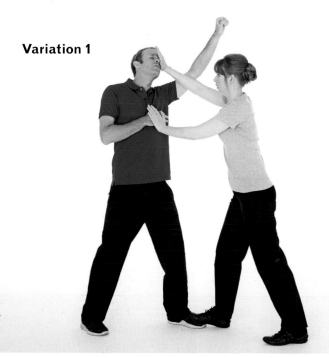
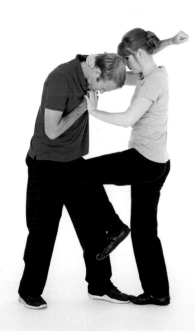

1. Step inside the opponent's punch, sliding your arm
along his arm and ending in a palm strike to the head,
jamming his arm against his chest.

2. Follow up by kneeing him in the groin.

Variation 2

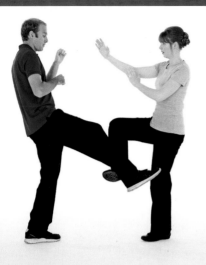

1. Raise your leg to defend against the kick.

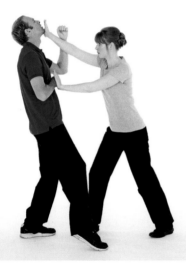

2. Jam his arm and palm-strike his head.

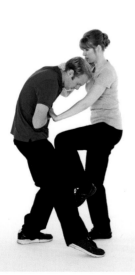

3. Follow up with a knee to the groin.

Variation 3

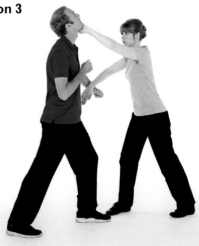

1. Intercept the body punch while simultaneously palm-striking the head.

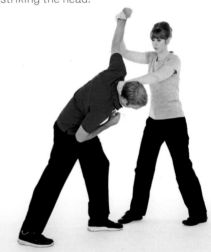

2. Use circular force to raise his arm and lower his head.

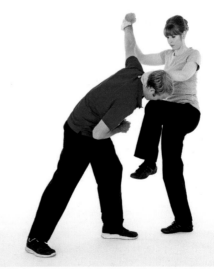

3. Follow up by kneeing him in the head.

Step Back to Ride the Tiger

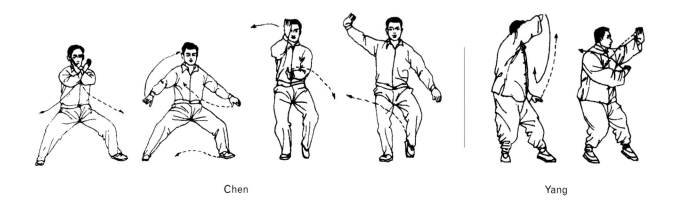

Chen   Yang

Variation 1

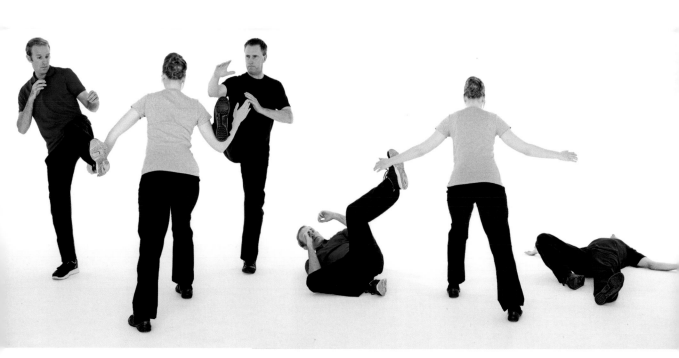

1. Step back and scoop the opponents' kicks.

2. Continue to raise their legs as you step forward and throw them to the ground.

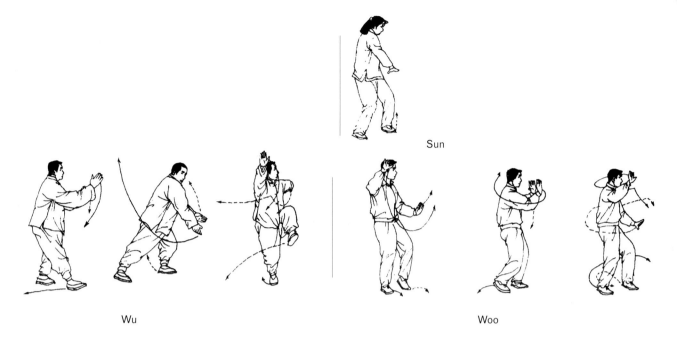

Sun

Wu

Woo

Variation 2

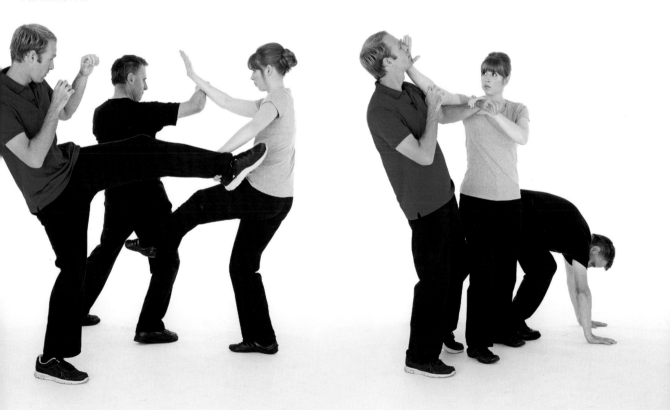

1. Step back slightly to intercept a kick and a punch. Kick the puncher's knee joint.

2. Turn and palm-strike the other opponent.

Draw the Bow to Shoot the Tiger

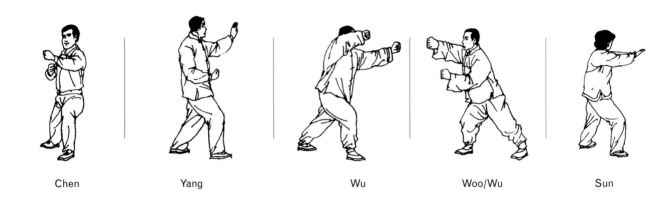

Chen   Yang   Wu   Woo/Wu   Sun

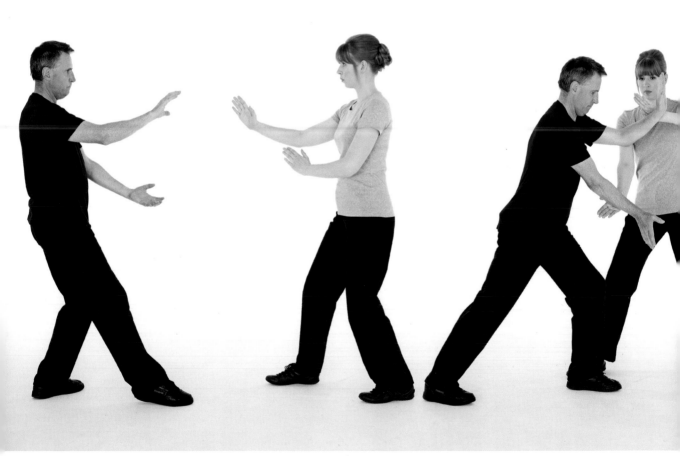

1. Face your hard-style opponent.

2. Evade and sweep aside his double palm strike.

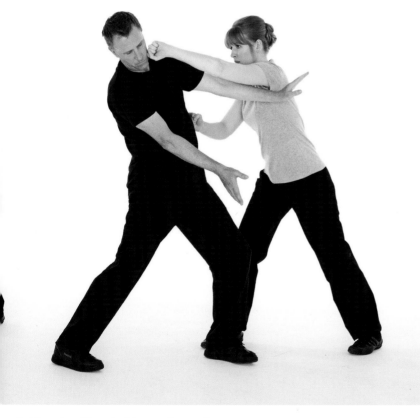

3. Move in with a double punch counter.

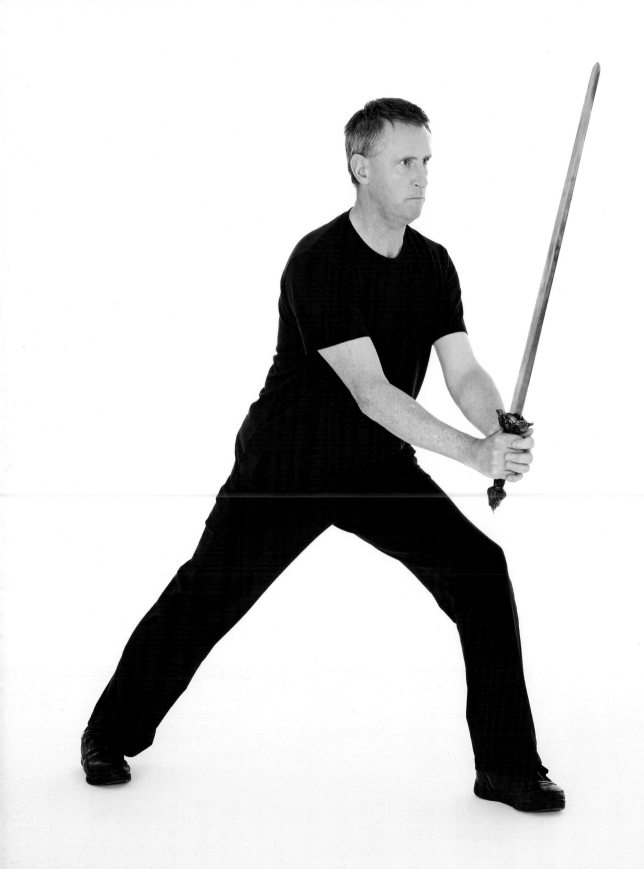

9 Have Sword, Will Travel

My old master mainly taught at his apartment or on the rooftop of his apartment building in Hong Kong and later at Tai Chi Heights on the outskirts of his village in China. I live in London, but I spend more than one third of the year outside the UK. I'm very fortunate in working with terrific people all over the world. Sometimes they come to stay with me, sometimes I go to them. My students are my teachers now.

Nowadays there is more access to Tai Chi tuition than ever before. In this chapter we'll look at how Tai Chi is taught and learned.

Teaching and Learning

Confucius was China's greatest teacher and many of his thoughts are still pertinent today.

'The superior man acts before he speaks and later speaks in accord with his actions.' In Chinese martial arts, including Tai Chi, the first thing is to do it, not talk about doing it.

'Learning without thought is a waste of time; thought without learning is dangerous.'

There are plenty of examples of both these extremes, especially on Internet Tai Chi groups. I recently read some posts by a couple of loquacious nerds who obviously had limited Tai Chi knowledge and even less knowledge of Chinese. I was appalled that they should be spreading this disinformation.

'When you know something, admit you know it; when you don't know it, admit you don't.'

This is a bit different from Laozi's 'Those who speak don't know; those who know don't speak.' The Internet nerd rarely possesses the nobility to follow this advice.

'Rotten wood can't be carved.'

The Song of the 13 Tactics states, 'In the attainment of perfection, don't waste Kung Fu (effort); carve and carve again into the mind it should be on the waist.' If the student won't listen, there's little the Sifu can do.

Confucius was realistic about people's ability to learn:

'To those who are less than mediocre higher matters may not be spoken of.'

My Sifu held very similar views. I try to be more patient.

Students need to take some responsibility for themselves. According to Confucius, 'When I've presented one corner of a subject to anyone and he can't learn the other three from it, I don't repeat my lesson.'

Confucius was an itinerant teacher who wandered from place to place with his disciples looking for official advancement. He didn't get it. He did, however, learn about people and about life:

'When three of us are walking, there is me and my teachers. I'll identify their good points and follow them, their bad points and avoid them.'

Classes, Workshops, Seminars and Camps

Not everyone can take years out of their lives to live in the Far East and learn Chinese, not everyone has ready access to expert tuition, whether for reasons of distance or time, and yet many people want to study Tai Chi Chuan in depth, in all its aspects.

There are many kinds of training available to those who want to pursue their knowledge of Tai Chi Chuan. It's up to you to find out what works for you. Some tutors teach too little too slowly; some teach too much too quickly. Some are perfectionists in an imperfect world. Some believe that the best way of teaching is to try to convince students that they, the teachers, know absolutely everything about absolutely everything. Perhaps most students believe this about their Sifu anyway.

So What's the Difference?

Seminar is jargon from the academic world; a relatively informal meeting between lecturer and students where each presents his or her views or papers on a topic of study.

Workshop is also jargon, used in academia to refer to a brief intensive course. Though the terms seminar and workshop are sometimes used interchangeably, in the Tai Chi world workshops usually only last one day and are of 1–6 hours duration, whereas seminars are normally done over a weekend and involve 4–6 hours tuition per day.

My Tai Chi Sifu didn't really run classes. His Wu Guan (martial gym) was on the rooftop of an 11-storey building in the middle of Kowloon. When it rained, we trained in the small downstairs studio. Official training times were two hours in the morning and two hours in the evening, six days a week, but once he got to know you he didn't mind when you came. The atmosphere was informal and, much of the time, there was no structure to the training.

Sifu had bouts of enthusiasm when he'd get more involved, but often he just left us to it. Often, too, he'd go with us for a drink or snack after we'd finished training; he was a great raconteur.

He didn't give a seminar in the real sense until 1981 – after more than 40 years in martial arts. Why? It wasn't the way things were done. In the old days disciples met their Sifu on an almost daily basis, or invited him to spend a concerted period with them. In those days ordinary people were more conservative and less willing or able to travel than they are now. My Sifu was no fool. The seminars he subsequently gave were more than classes, but less than 'inside the door' training.

I look at Tai Chi seminars as part of the entertainment industry; the aim is to capture the interest of the students and only then to make them think. Proper teaching of concepts and technique requires not only that information is sent out, but also that it is both understood and acted upon. So it helps to have structure. When giving seminars and workshops, I often try to follow concept themes or teach sequential form applications, whereas in classes the training is more routine.

When I was doing a Postgraduate Diploma in Chinese at Ealing College, London, one of the students in my seminar group was having great difficulty with the text we were working on which described the 'Long March'. Finally, after three weeks of unequal struggle, Patrick told

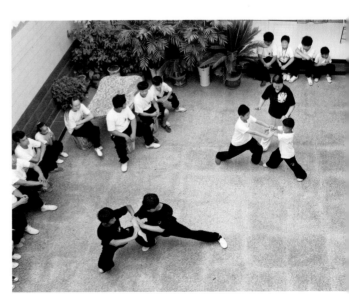

Right Pushing Hands class.

the tutor that he couldn't make head or tail of the text. It transpired that although Patrick had been reading the Chinese text from top to bottom, he had also been reading from left to right, instead of from right to left. For Patrick, Chinese was truly a Long March. There is no shortage of seminar-attending Patricks in the Tai Chi world.

There are now dozens of Tai Chi events all over the world and joint/multi-style seminars, often on a specific theme, are common. Seminars have also become a way of having contact with other instructors and other styles and breaking down barriers.

Camps

The Tai Chi camps I teach at are often residential and can involve outdoor training. They usually last at least three days. This gives me time to get to know people and them time to get to know me and one another, and helps to create a personal relationship akin to that between me and my Sifu. In particular it gives people the time to build up the courage to ask questions.

In 1980, I attended the Royal Hong Kong Police instructor training course, during which we were trained to instruct recruit inspectors. When teaching at Tai Chi camps I use the format I learned then: I ask the more experienced students to show or explain techniques or concepts; then, if anything is unclear or incorrect, we have a discussion and criticism session and try to find a better way.

In camps we cover Hand Form, Pushing Hands, self-defence applications and weapons. People who have met the basic requirements may do specialized training such as Neigong.

'Inside the Door'

In most classes teachers and students just get on with the training; there isn't time to cover techniques or concepts in depth. Instead, Chinese martial arts such as Tai Chi have 'inside the door' training, when the Sifu becomes a super tutor to the pupil, who becomes a disciple. Many things my Sifu taught me he never taught in any class, but on a one-to-one basis: inside the door. It is very difficult to teach in a detailed way in a normal class. Stupid or lazy students don't understand; clever but unpleasant people – well, teacher isn't too keen on teaching them.

I first started giving workshops and seminars back in 1984. Now I do dozens every year. It gives me direct contact with second and third generation students in the UK and abroad. It enables me to meet their teachers regularly to improve their standards, too. Some subsequently fall by the wayside, some move on to become certificated teachers, helping in their turn to pass

on the art. In my school, those who are interested may if they wish be awarded a training or instructor's certificate. Some tutors operate a system where certificates need to be renewed yearly by mandatory attendance at workshops; that has always seemed a bit greedy to me.

Private Tuition

When I was at high school, I had tutors for French and mathematics and it certainly made a difference. My time is limited and I value it, so I prefer to give private lessons to small groups, including residential groups working on particular themes, rather than working with just one person. This makes tuition cheaper for the student and is a better use of my time, too.

Confucius once observed, 'I've never refused instruction to anyone.'

I run open classes, seminars and camps; all are welcome. Because people aren't the same, I won't treat them the same. Private tuition is a whole different story and when the chemistry is wrong with someone, I won't work with them. Life is too short.

Oral Transmission

Learning in a class is important, attending seminars is important, but to really understand a Tai Chi system there is no substitute for direct contact with a tutor whether through private lessons or accompanying him on trips to martial arts events. Even if you're not receiving secrets, you need personal attention and detailed instruction if you really want to understand what you're doing.

In *The Song of the 13 Tactics* it is written, 'If you are to enter the door and be led along the path, oral instruction is necessary.'

In other words there are many things that are not written down, that are not taught in open classes, that can't just be downloaded from the Internet. This type of teaching is vital for anyone who wants to achieve anything approaching mastery. Over many years I accompanied my Sifu to Singapore, Malaysia, China, Australia and other places. I often shared a room with him. In many ways he treated me like a son; in many ways I treated him like a father. These experiences were far more instructive than any formal instruction I received.

Sometimes Tai Chi tutors ask for what seems like a lot of money, whether for classes, for seminars or for private lessons. Remember, though, that what you are paying for, if you have an honest and able teacher, is not the work of one or two hours, but the knowledge of a lifetime.

American Tai Chi and Bagua teacher Aarvo Tucker once related how at different times he lived with both his Tai Chi master and his Bagua master and actually taught for the latter in Taiwan. In a similar way, I often slept at my Sifu's place and he would get me to show Pushing Hands and fighting applications to his sons. As foreigners we were without family ties in the Far East – we had left home, friends and family to learn the art. We grew close to our teachers because we gave everything for the art. We went eating with them, drinking with them and socializing also.

A good account of this type of life, though in an Aikido setting, is given in Robert Twigger's book *Angry White Pyjamas*. Through this type of direct personal contact, listening to and watching your teacher, inevitably you learn and perceive things that you never could by just attending classes a few times a week. However, many people see, but few observe and fewer still are able to analyse or synthesize these observations. A simple example. One of my senior students who had many times seen me put students through the Tai Chi ritual initiation ceremony attempted to help me at one such ceremony by lighting the joss sticks; he lit the wrong end.

As Robert Twigger points out, it is considered an honour to be selected as the master's Uke (Japanese for the person on whom the technique is performed), because only in this way can you learn the feel of the technique at a high level. The greater the pain, the greater the honour.

Because of this close contact between earlier masters and non-family members, including non-Chinese, famous Tai Chi families have been forced to invent more secrets, to make more changes in the Tai Chi which they teach, though not necessarily the Tai Chi they practise. They want it back, but it's too late. I strongly suspect that in some cases the Tai Chi Chuan of the famous families has changed even more than the Tai Chi outside the families, and not always for the better.

Below Demonstrating San Shou against two opponents at my Black Sea Camp in Bulgaria.

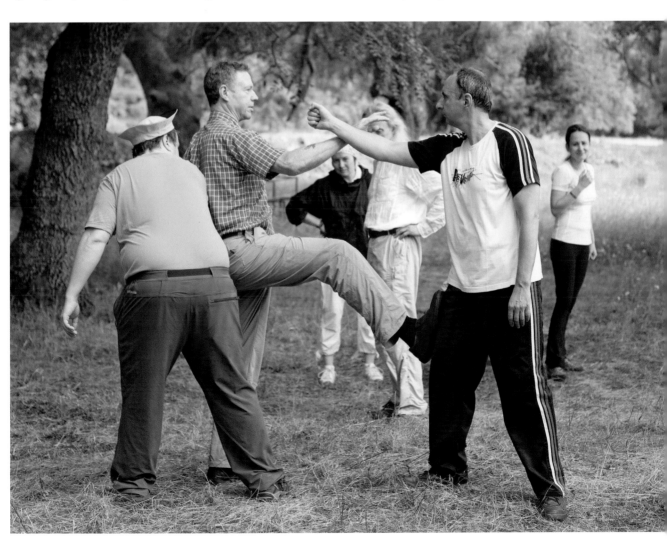

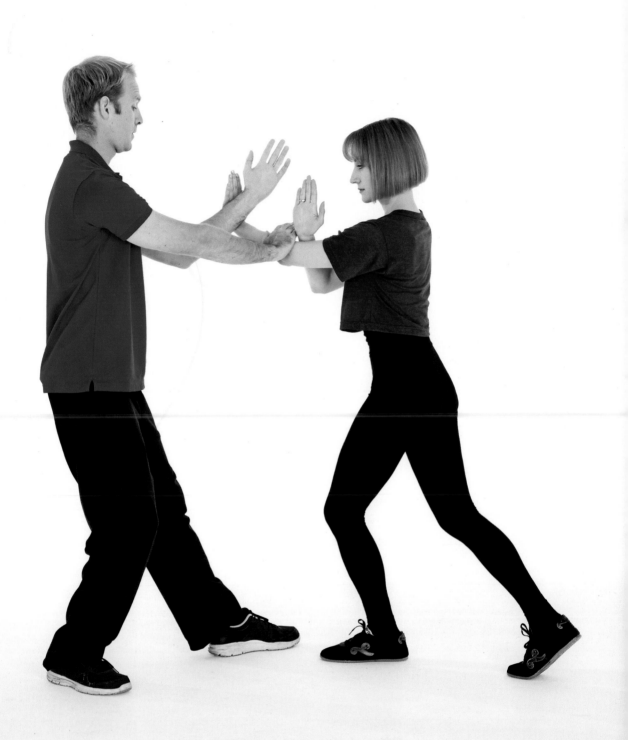

10 Specialist Tuition

The subject of specialist tuition is rarely
addressed in Tai Chi books; not every
Tai Chi teacher is a Renaissance man or
woman. Here we are going to look at areas
of tuition that won't be familiar to even
some of the more experienced Tai Chi tutors.
We'll begin by covering the different aspects
of teaching self-defence.

Tai Chi Tutors and Self-Defence

Most Tai Chi tutors have never hit anybody or been hit by anybody. They've never used the Tai Chi they've practised so assiduously in a real fight. No matter how good you are in sparring or practising applications, once you enter the house of pain, the game changes.

There are many different types of self-defence. In a military context, it may be necessary to render the enemy unconscious or even dead. Police and security staff often use 'control and restraint' to pacify, remove or arrest members of the public. My old student, Dr Don Welikele, who has been my medical adviser for this book, said he had encountered similar problems in Accident and Emergency, where sometimes up to six staff members were needed to handle a violent patient without resorting to striking him. Kickboxing and arts such as Tae Kwon Do, with their emphasis on striking, are particularly unsuitable for this type of encounter.

When I attended the Royal Hong Kong Police Training School back in 1975, George Button, the Chief Physical Training Instructor, based his self-defence course mainly on Aikido and Judo moves, though he had also trained in Tai Chi. Tai Chi offers control of an opponent through Pushing Hands skills and Qin Na/Seizing and Holding; for police and security, striking the opponent is normally a last resort. In my nine years' police service, including time as a Detective Inspector in charge of an investigation team and seven months in command of the Kowloon Regional Vice Squad, I made many hundreds of arrests and found the Tai Chi techniques I had learned to be highly practical.

Before we begin, let's make a few things clear. Firstly, if you're going to punch someone, be aware that you can easily damage your knuckles on the hard bones in the opponent's face. For this reason, my dad, who was a doctor in a rough area of Glasgow, would often wear a knuckleduster when making house calls late at night.

Women's legs are proportionately stronger in relation to their arms than are men's, so kicks, stamps and knee strikes are recommended for them. Palm strikes, finger thrusts, chops and elbow strikes to vital points are good, too. Punches are fine also, against soft tissue like the groin, the nose and the kidneys.

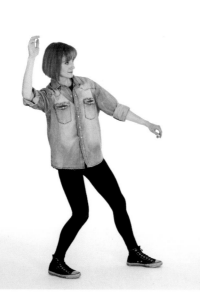 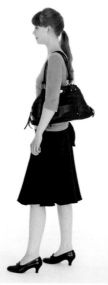

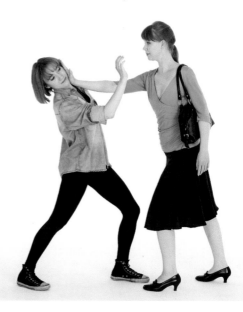

1. The opponent (left) starts to move.

2. The victim moves first, stepping in with a pre-emptive palm strike.

The main aim of a man who gets into a fight is usually to win, to beat his attacker. Women are usually more sensible and try to avoid a fight in the first place. If attacked, most women don't want to get into a fist fight or wrestling match against a bigger, stronger opponent. Their aim is to do enough to get away from the scene of the trouble to a place of safety. A useful additional skill is to be able to use whatever is at hand as a weapon. This is why I chose a medium-sized female Tai Chi tutor to demonstrate the Tai Chi-based self-defence moves, some involving the use of weapon techniques, in this book.

The attacks we are trying to counter may vary in gravity from harassment to serious assault.

Our response, if we are attacked, should be both within the law and practical. We should apply only reasonable force. It may be reasonable for a small woman to use a knife to defend herself against a large man. It is unlikely to be considered reasonable force if the large man is holding the knife to defend himself against the small woman.

Once the threat to us is over, our defence should cease too; we are not entitled to beat up an aggressor. It isn't necessary for an opponent to actually hit or grab us before we can react; a reasonable apprehension that they intend to do so is enough (see left). Usually there is some kind of a building up of aggression before we arrive at a self-defence situation.

For some years in the 1990s I ran Management of Aggression courses for trainee security guards and hospital staff. I taught them some transactional analysis and showed them how to use body language to control potentially aggressive situations so as to prevent the aggression becoming physical.

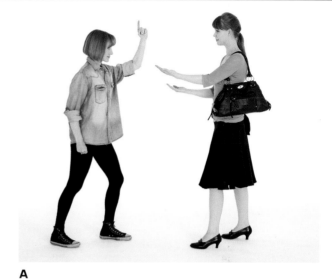

A

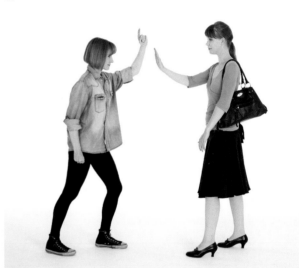

B

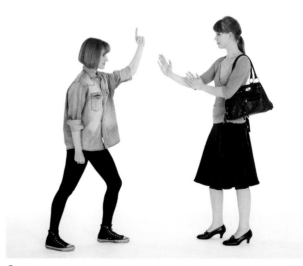

C

A The oponent (left) is using aggressive body language; the victim tries to defuse the situation by using the open palm gesture to show sincerity, but at the same time the arms are acting as a guard, controlling the distance.

B The victim (left) is using more commanding body language; the palm down gesture is used by police and security personnel to keep people at a distance or control traffic etc.

C The victim's response to her opponent's threatening gestures is to adopt a Seven Star Guard, which also looks aggressive.

The palm-down gesture is very assertive – police and security staff often use it to stop people in their tracks. The open-palm gesture is much more friendly and is used by conmen and politicians to give the impression that they are honest and open. Both these gestures are useful alternatives to a clenched-fist, boxing type of guard. In a clenched-fist guard, unless you are very skilled indeed, you are mainly going to be punching – not an ideal scenario for our medium-sized female doing Tai Chi-based self-defence. Note how both the palm-down and the open-palm gestures can be used like a Tai Chi Seven Star guard to control the distance between the victim and her aggressor.

You will see that in all the victim's encounters with her aggressor, she plays the percentages, largely avoiding the use of force against force and mainly employing simple and direct techniques to access the aggressor's vital points and buy the time to escape (vital points include the eyes, nose, ears, temples, throat, solar plexus, floating ribs, kidneys, hands and fingers, and knee joints). This is important; as soon as the aggressor is clearly out of action and there is an opportunity to leave, you should do so immediately. You are not the police. Personal safety comes first.

With any kind of self-defence, there are three key factors. The first is distance. The Canon of Tai Chi Chuan states, 'When he advances, the distance seems surpassingly long; when he retreats, the distance seems surpassingly short.' Once you have evaded an attack, the distance will decide what counter is most suitable.

The next is timing. The Canon of Tai Chi Chuan says, 'If the opponent's actions are swift, then my response is swift. If the opponent's actions are slow, then I slowly follow them.' Moving too slowly or too early can get you into a whole lot of trouble.

Finally there is the matter of the angles of attack and defence. According to An Interpretation of the Practice of the 13 Tactics, 'When standing, the body should be centrally correct and at ease to deal with attacks from the eight directions.' Note how our heroine makes extensive use of footwork to change the angle, generate momentum and make her techniques more effective. Two of the key methods of developing skill in achieving correct distance, timing and posture are Seven Stars and Nine Palace Step pushing hands drills (see right).

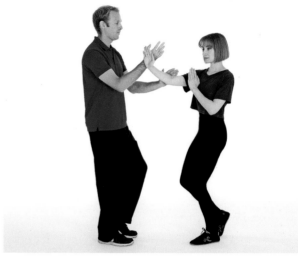

1a. Seven Star Step Pushing Hands: She steps with the left foot and pushes with the right hand while he steps back with the right foot and diverts her push.

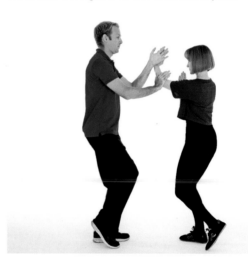

1b. They do the same movements, but in reverse.

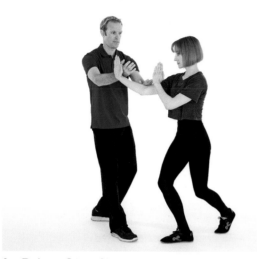

2a. Palace Step. She steps with the right foot and pushes with the right hand which he intercepts and diverts

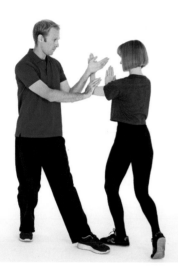

2b. They do the same movements, but in reverse.

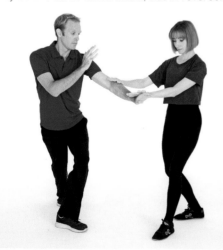

2c. Now it's his turn to push.

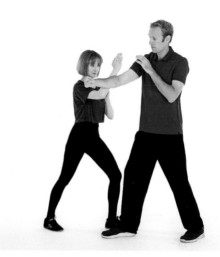

3a. She evades the punch.

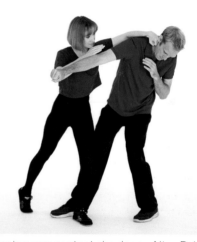

3b. Keeping arm contact she does a Nine Palace Step with her left foot as she punches.

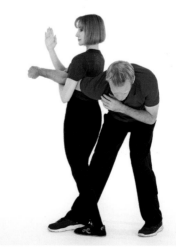

3c. She spins, trapping his arm.

Many people these days talk about Mixed Martial Arts as if it's something new; it's not. Tai Chi is versatile in that its concepts and techniques can be applied in a wide variety of situations; unfortunately many Tai Chi tutors are not proficient in the self-defence aspect, though they may know some applications. I often tell students that there are no techniques in Tai Chi. Through practice under the instruction of a competent tutor, a student will refine his technique and develop the ability to express the key Yin/Yang concept of change without even thinking about it. This stage is beyond technique.

Only a few core techniques are shown here; there are many other possibilities. It's better to be able to do a few things well than many things badly.

Womens' self-defence through Tai Chi is a subject in its own right. Women are different from men: often with long hair, smaller hands and with proportionately stronger legs. Women also dress differently from men in dresses, skirts, heeled shoes and often carry a handbag. The corollary of this is that they will face different situations and use different counters than a man would. Few Tai Chi books deal with self-defence; as for those that do, it is almost unheard of for a Tai Chi book to feature ladies using the Yin/Yang duality of Tai Chi for self-defence. As demonstrated here, this book has now changed that sad state of affairs. The techniques on pages 206–213 all use Tai Chi concepts to deal with a variety of different scenarios, including using a ladies' umbrella to mimic Tai Chi sword techniques.

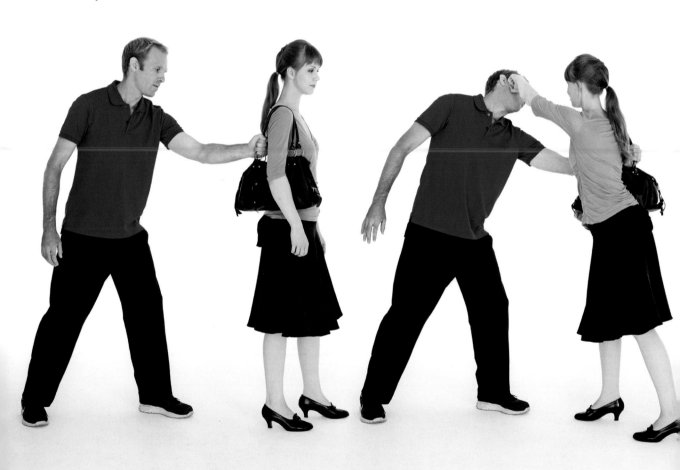

1. The attacker grabs the victim's bag from behind.

2. Going with the pull she turns and hits him in the face.

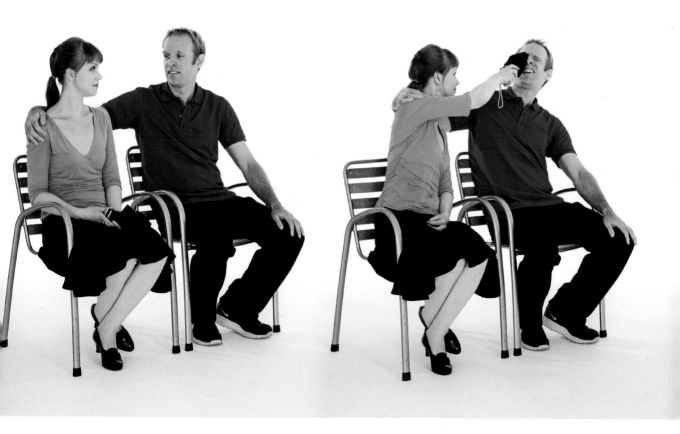

1. This unwanted advance is technically an assault.

2. She goes with the pull and counters it by hitting him in the face with her umbrella.

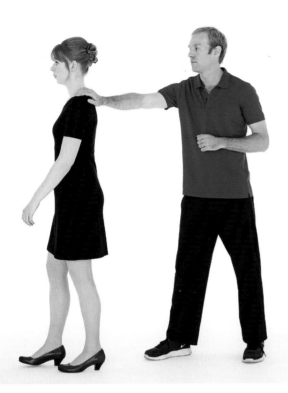
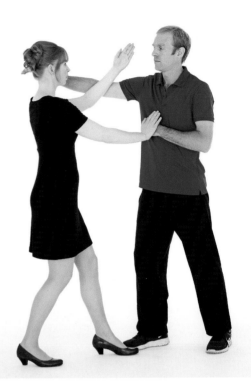

1. The attacker grabs the victim's shoulder.

2. Following his force she spins and controls his arms.

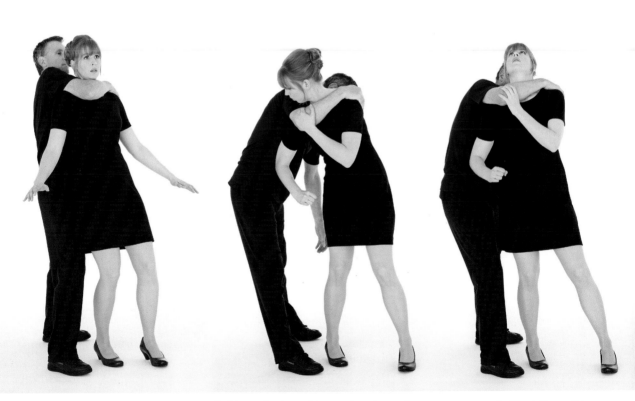

1. The attacker grabs the victim from behind.

2. She pulls down his arm to release the pressure and hits him with an elbow to the ribs.

3. She follows this up with a head butt.

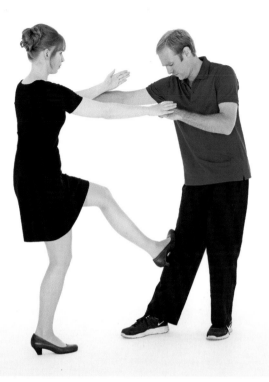

3. She stamps at his knee joint.

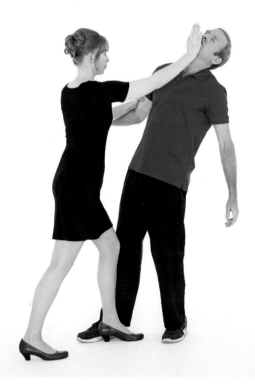

4. She follows up with a palm strike.

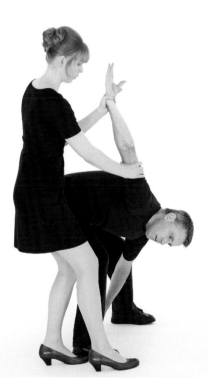

4. She twists out of the hold and locks his arm.

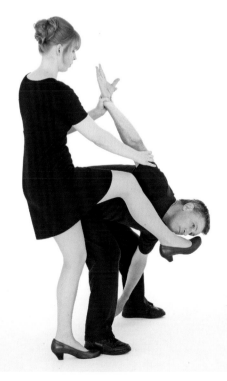

5. She counters with a kick.

Tai Chi and Competitions

When I started practising Tai Chi, my Sifu had many skilful and experienced Chinese students who enjoyed every aspect of the art, but the only outlet for those interested in competing was Chinese full-contact fighting. Over the years this has changed.

Now there are competitions for Hand Form, Weapon Forms, Group Forms and two-person sets (with and without weapons), Junior Forms, Senior Forms, Beginner, Intermediate and Open Forms (with and without weapons). There is competition in Fixed Step, Restricted Step or Moving Step Pushing Hands and Shuai Jiao/ Chinese wrestling with different weight divisions. Finally, there is Chinese full-contact fighting. I started the annual British Open Tai Chi Championships in 1989 and it is the longest running TaI Chi competition in Europe.

Students of mine have taken part in all these types of competition over the years with a high degree of success. For a lot of people competition provides a motivation and focus for their training and becomes a test for their skills under pressure. Tai Chi competition isn't for everyone, but it does have its good points.

On the negative side, some competitors, especially those doing modern competition forms, often develop back and joint problems because they over-extend in order to impress the judges. Competition in Pushing Hands and full contact can result in a whole range of injuries. It is the responsibility of the Tai Chi tutor to prepare his students properly.

Forms Competition

In 1991 at the Third British Open Tai Chi Championships, I introduced rules for forms competition with ten judging criteria for Hand Form and ten for Weapon Forms. These criteria will mostly be familiar to you from other sections of the book. They are largely self-explanatory and not specific to any one style.

Criteria for Hand Form
1. Correct posture
2. Correct stance
3. Distinguishing Yin and Yang
4. Intent and focus
5. Coordination
6. Smooth transitions between techniques
7. Balanced turning and stepping
8. Softness and relaxation of the body
9. Aesthetic appearance
10. Martial spirit

Criteria for Weapon Forms
1. Correct posture
2. Correct stance
3. Distinguishing Yin and Yang
4. Intent and focus
5. Harmony between body and weapon
6. Correct use of Jin
7. Balance and agility
8. Control of weapon
9. Aesthetic appearance
10. Martial spirit

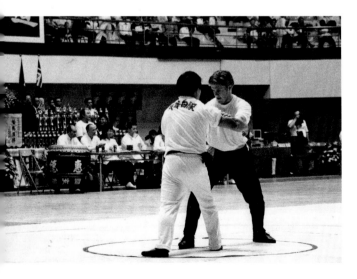

Left Chung Hwa Tai Chi Cup, Taiwan, 1990. My student Steve Wooster (UK) pushing hands against a Taiwanese opponent.

The main object of forms competition is not just to do the form correctly, but to impress the judges with aesthetic appearance and martial spirit. I therefore coach students to exaggerate the contrasts of expand and contract, rise and sink and so on, and where appropriate to use broken rhythm and 'freeze frame' techniques to make the form more lively.

The other key to preparing for forms competitions is repetition of the form. I once interviewed well-respected British international Tai Chi competitors Simon Watson and Chew Yeen Lawes. They told me that in their team training sessions they'd do 20 non-stop repetitions of the 42-step competition form, each repetition taking 5–6 minutes.

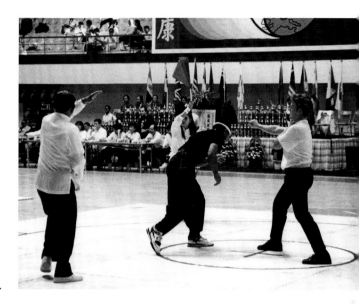

Right My student Steve Wooster defeating one of the top American competitors.
Below The British team at the 1990 Chung Hwa Tai Chi cup in Taiwan. Dan Docherty (wearing a tie) standing between trophy winner Steve Wooster and well-known British sifu, Nigel Sutton.

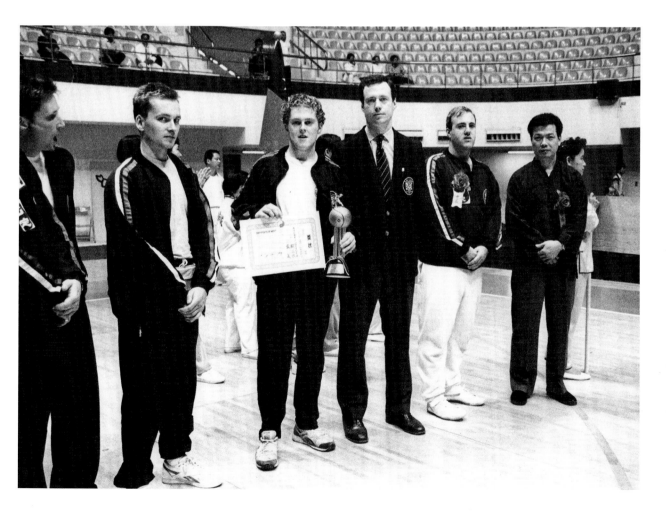

Pushing Hands and Shuai Jiao Competition

Pushing Hands events can be Fixed Step, Restricted Step or Moving Step.

In Fixed Step, competitors' feet need to stay in the same place: the object is to unbalance the opponent by pulling, pushing and so on, so that his feet move.

Restricted Step is similar to fixed, but limited foot movement is allowed.

In Moving Step, competitors can move their feet freely, normally within a designated area as they try to unbalance one another or force one another out of the area. Sometimes, in addition to pushing and pulling, throwing, sweeping and locking are allowed too.

Shuai Jiao competition is somewhat similar to Judo; it involves throwing, sweeping and locking as well as grabbing the opponent's jacket.

In Pushing Hands competitions, irrespective of the weight category, victory tends to go to the more skilful competitor. But when stamina goes, technique goes; when technique goes, you are likely to be defeated.

It is understandable if your student loses to a more skilful competitor, but it is not acceptable if he loses because he lacks stamina. This means that in addition to the normal Pushing Hands skill training, adequate conditioning training is also necessary.

In 1991, I took a British team to Hong Kong for an international Pushing Hands tournament. The Guangdong province champions were taking part. I talked to their coach, who told me his charges were all in their twenties and didn't practise Tai Chi Forms.

Instead, they went running, lifted weights and practised competition Pushing Hands. Only my best students could beat these professional Chinese athletes.

Full Contact

Chinese full-contact fighting is referred to as San Shou/Scattering Hands, Guoshu/National Art and Lei Tai/Striking Platform.

Nowadays full-contact fighters wear helmets, heavy gloves and groin and shin protection. Traditionally fights are on a raised platform, but there are no ropes as in a boxing ring; I've seen fighters fall off and break arms and legs. I was kicked off the platform only once, but managed to roll with it. Permitted techniques include kicks and punches to the head and body, throws, sweeps and locks. Fights are normally over three two-minute rounds.

As with training for Pushing Hands and Shuai Jiao, for full-contact fighters conditioning training is essential – for at least three months before the competition, around two hours a day, every day. I'm still amazed by some would-be masters who obviously haven't prepared their students for a full-contact fight. It's irresponsible and unprofessional. As my old police drill and musketry instructor Gus To still likes to say, 'Failing to plan is planning to fail.'

Full contact fighting is dangerous. Many years ago in Hong Kong, I was one of the judges in a competition where a 17-year-old boy was killed by a roundhouse kick to the neck. I knew the boy who killed him. He was also just 17 years old.

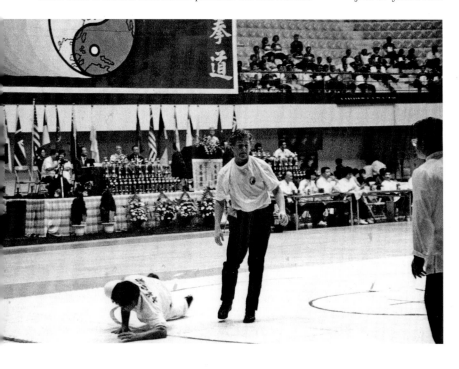

Left Steve Wooster after throwing his Taiwanese opponent to the ground.

Judging and Refereeing

I've run courses in judging and refereeing forms, Pushing Hands and Chinese full-contact competitions in Britain, Sweden, France, Hungary, Ukraine, Ireland, Bulgaria and Denmark.

It's easier to judge forms than to referee, because you have time to reflect and discuss. Refereeing takes a lot of concentration and requires the ability to make snap decisions under pressure. For forms competitions, normally it's a good idea to have a judges' meeting beforehand to discuss how competitors are going to be assessed. The first competitor gives you the standard. Judging Tai Chi forms will improve your ability to understand what makes good Tai Chi and what doesn't and will improve your game as a Tai Chi tutor and practitioner.

Competitors deserve fairness and respect. Many have trained for months, travelled a long way and paid their entry fees.

Made in Taiwan

Back in 1994, Huang Jifu, Vice Chairman of the British Council of Chinese Martial Arts, was the team leader. Dick Watson and I were the coaches for a squad of 20 which went with us to Taiwan for the Second Chung Hua Cup International Tal Chi Chuan Tournament. I'd been with three of my students to the First Chung Hua Cup, so I had an idea what to expect.

I quote from the tournament regulations: 'Purpose: Owing to expend (sic) Chinese culture, promote the acknowledge of Tai Chi Chuan, encourage the health of human being, as well as improving and learning the technical of Tai Chi Chuan.' Despite the faulty English, I think the gist is clear.

This tournament failed to achieve any of these noble purposes.

The travel guide to Taiwan thoughtfully provided by the Free China Centre told us, 'Try never to shout or lose your temper. Always stay calm and cool. Be modest and respectful, the more so with someone older or more senior.'

Halfway through the first day of competition, I had metamorphosed from an urbane, courteous Dr Jekyll into a raging, slavering Mr Hyde. As Jifu remarked, even Dick Watson, normally the most mild-mannered and pleasant of people, was seething. Contest after contest went against us, despite our protests.

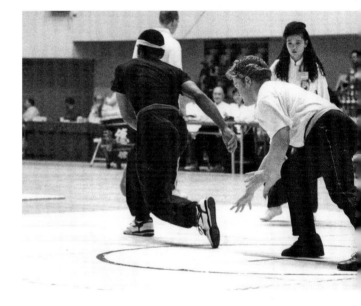

Above Steve Wooster unbalancing an American opponent.

In one contest, the Taiwanese opponent was so well beaten that he was shaking his head when time was called. Nevertheless he got the decision. Jifu made a protest. The Taiwanese judges and organizers smiled at us, shook our hands and said nice things.

The referee of the next contest seemed even worse, so I walked on and stopped the contest. I told the chief judge and his retinue that if they were incapable of judging and refereeing properly, we could do it for them. The judges were visibly shaken and obviously unused to being harangued in Mandarin by a 1.85m, 90kg (6ft 1in, 200lb) Scots guy. However, organizers came over and smiled and said more nice things. I let it continue.

When the time came, we thought our boy had won narrowly, but the judges gave it to the Taiwanese, by 25–8; this was the last straw. Our team was a good one, but there was little point in continuing, so we withdrew. I felt sorry for those who had been wronged, sorry for those who had fought their way through to the semi-finals, sorry for those who hadn't had the chance to compete.

They sent the President of the Taiwan International Tai Chi Chuan Federation (and Jifu's Tai Chi uncle) to shake hands with me and smooth things over. I refused to shake hands with him and told them that they had spoken many beautiful words but very few true ones.

Later, at the party, Jifu came up and said that he'd been told that his uncle, the President, wanted to give personal presents to him and to me and would I go up onto the stage to accept. I refused, but said that in view of his being in the same Tai Chi family I understood that it was necessary for him to accept. He didn't get the chance. The Taiwanese persuaded one of our team members to go up and sing and, at the end of a rendition of 'Stand by Me', they made an announcement in Mandarin that they were presenting a framed portrait to the British team – which they duly did, with smiles, clapping and photographs.

When our team member came down from the stage I asked to look at the portrait. I took it over to the bleachers and started to smash it on the metal railings. The first crash got their attention; after the second I flung it on the floor. There was a stunned silence followed by an angry outcry.

Only now do I understand what happened. If you have strong views on a subject such as religion, such as politics, such as martial arts, it is common to reject any evidence that runs contrary to those views, no matter how strong the evidence might be. As far as those Taiwanese officials were concerned, they are Chinese and Tai Chi is a Chinese art. Chinese people are best at Tai Chi. Chinese cannot be bested by foreigners in Tai Chi competition, so even if it seems to be happening it isn't happening. This world view seems less prevalent in Hong Kong and China. In both places I have seen the rules fairly applied and my students have competed successfully.

To Chinese people 'face' is extremely important, so rejecting their present was the most effective way to make a non-violent protest. I heard recently that they still remember me, though 20 years have passed. But I learned something from the experience.

I've never been back.

Dutch Treat

The Executive Committee of the Taijiquan and Qigong Federation for Europe (TCFE) unanimously accepted the bid of the Dutch Tai Chi Stichting to run the first TCFE Tai Chi Championships in Utrecht in the Netherlands in 2000. Though I was the other obvious candidate (I was TCFE Vice President at the time), I didn't make a bid, guessing there'd be all kinds of trouble organizing the first such event and firmly believing the old British Army adage, 'Never volunteer for anything.'

Prior to the TCFE event I was a judge at the Danish Open Tai Chi Championships. It was low key and well organized, but one thing after another went wrong. One well-known competitor dropped his spear, but was given first place in the spear event. Another made a mistake in his form, stopped, began all over again and was still awarded a medal. The awards were made with good intentions, but it was wrong, unprofessional and unacceptable.

I realized that if nothing was done the TCFE event would be a disaster. I tried to intervene by sending emails to the TCFE's Dutch President, who was not a friend, but a man I respected. The only reply was that there could be no meeting and the rules could not be changed.

I invoked the TCFE statutes so that an Emergency General Meeting had to be held. The President began the meeting by saying that the chief Pushing Hands referee, Rob Volke, wished to read a statement. Rob stood up and said, 'If the meeting tries to change the rules, all the referees will walk out.'

I realized then what was going on. I knew Rob to be a sincere person, so I asked him, 'So, Rob, are you telling us that in an international competition only Dutch people are going to be referees?'

To a room full of Scandinavians, Irish, Russians, French, Bulgarians and more, he said yes. I asked him if he was seriously suggesting that, in the whole of Europe, only the Dutch knew how to referee. It was then agreed that to get things under way, the Dutch would referee the first few contests of the tournament, then we'd change the officials.

The Pushing Hands rules stated that if the referee thought a push that unbalanced a competitor to be a good one, he could award four points; if it was an ordinary push he'd award one point. Try those tricks in international soccer and see where it gets you.

We changed the rules. No-one walked out. On the final night, the Dutch thanked me and treated me to dinner. I kid you not.

Land of the Litigant

These are my reminiscences from the 1993 US National Chinese Martial Arts Championships in Orlando, Florida, home of Disney World.

I saw back flips in the Traditional Spear Form event. I saw people spin the Spear; I saw them throwing it in the air and catching it behind them; I saw them whacking the carpet with it; I saw them throw it, catch it and do the splits. Doc Fai Wong's son even spun it round his legs and dropped it. And the crowd – composed almost entirely of fellow competitors – went crazy every time anyone did any of these things.

The competitors were good gymnasts. They were good jugglers. They were good acrobats. I don't know whether or not they were good weapons men, because for the most part they weren't using the Spear as a weapon. In all the Traditional Form events it was the same story. The reason was obvious. The audience had been brought up on a diet of Jackie Chan movies.

I was told that the highly technical Pushing Hands rules were designed to prevent litigation in the event of injury. Sam Masich from Canada, a former champion, told me that he didn't favour these rules himself and indeed he had to be corrected on their implementation on a number of occasions. With a few exceptions the judges were scrupulously fair and strict in their interpretation of the rules. It was the rules themselves that were questionable.

Marvin Smallheiser of *Tai Chi* magazine was there. I've corresponded with him for some years and I know that he is a very open person with a genuine desire to promote all aspects of Tai Chi in his magazine, even when he himself doesn't agree with a particular approach. He is a real gentleman.

One man not doing back flips was Wong Tat Mau, one of the leading Chinese martial arts instructors in the USA. I hadn't seen him for about 15 years. In 1976 we were both members of the Hong Kong full-contact Kung Fu team which fought in the Fourth Southeast Asian Martial Arts Championships in Singapore. He now runs the biggest Chinese martial arts tournament in America.

We had a chat about the full-contact event which, apart from some of the masters' demos, was one of the few instances of genuine Chinese Kung Fu, as opposed to modern Wu Shu. There was minimal interference from the officials. Tat Mau agreed with me that, at 450g (16oz), the gloves were too big, but this was to protect the organizers from the risk of being sued by injured participants.

I also managed to have a chat with Jeff Bolt, the tournament organizer. He must be congratulated for getting so many prominent martial artists together in one place for four days and getting them to cooperate with one another. He told me that there were plans to make the event shorter. I agreed that this would be a good move as it got very tedious at times – particularly during the numerous time-outs the judges took to discuss the rules.

I brought back some new ideas, such as having Beginner and Intermediate Form events, and made rule changes which favour a more physical Pushing Hands approach.

Competition Round-up

In general Tai Chi Pushing Hands competitions are less popular now than they were in their heyday of the 1990s – numbers haven't increased much since then. In addition to the places I've mentioned, Tai Chi competitions are/ have been held in Australia, Austria, Belgium, Canada, Germany, Italy, Bulgaria, Hungary, Romania, Latvia, Sweden and Switzerland. The rules may vary somewhat, but generally success goes to the better prepared and more skilled competitors.

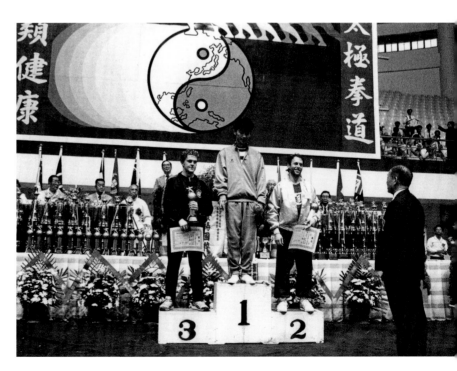

Right Chung Hwa Cup awards ceremony, 1990.

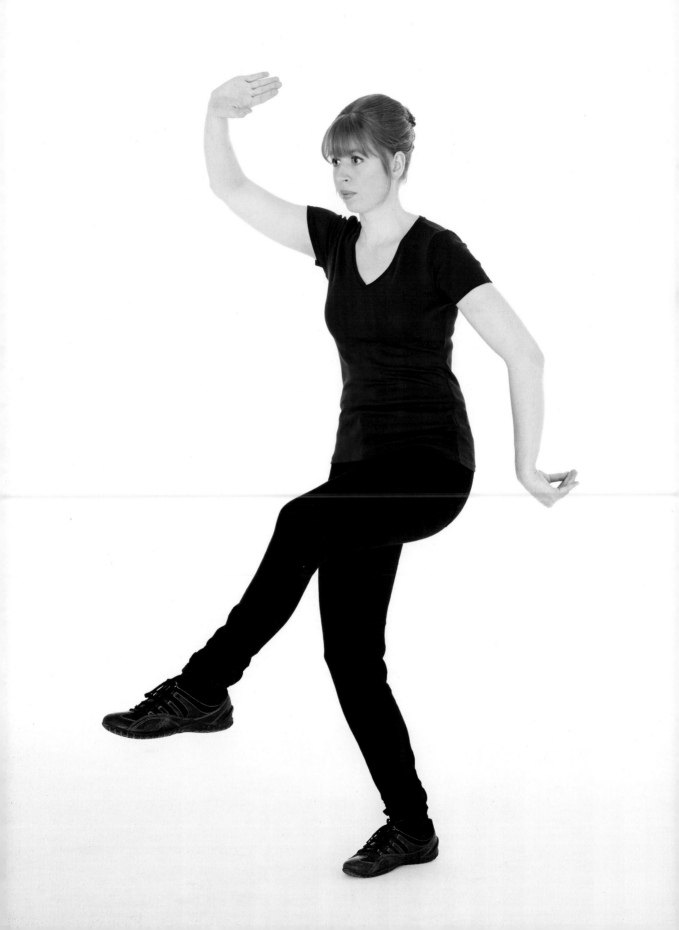

11 The Reality of Oneness

The essential paradigm of Tai Chi is the reality of oneness. Yin and Yang are not two separate things; they are two aspects of one thing and there is Yin in Yang and Yang in Yin.

This final section of this book deals with the professional aspects of being a Tai Chi tutor, with a look at different countries.

We'll talk about giving and receiving different types of tuition such as coaching for competition (whether as a judge, competitor or coach); private and 'inside the door' tuition; teaching the old and the young, and giving relevant self-defence training to the target audience, whether they be male or female. We'll also review some interesting and useful books for the hard-core enthusiast.

Knowledge of a Lifetime

In many places, including the UK, anyone at all can and often does set themselves up as a Tai Chi tutor. There are no official requirements to be a member of or certified by a professional body. There are no requirements at all. Even if there were, in the end things come down to the knowledge and ability of each individual tutor.

James Abbott McNeill Whistler, the great Impressionist painter and etcher, was a contemporary and verbal sparring partner of Oscar Wilde. John Ruskin, Professor of Art at Oxford University, once described one of Whistler's paintings as the first example he had seen of a coxcomb throwing a pot of paint in the public's face and demanding the sum of 200 guineas for the privilege. Whistler sued for libel. In his book *The Gentle Art of Making Enemies*, Whistler recalls Ruskin's lawyer asking how long it took him to paint the *Nocturne in Black and Gold – The Falling Rocket*. Whistler replied that it probably took two days. The lawyer followed up with the charge that, for the work of two days, Whistler was demanding the outrageous sum of 200 guineas. Whistler replied, 'Not for the work of one or two days; for the knowledge of a lifetime.' Whistler won the case and was awarded a farthing in damages.

In the Tai Chi world, if the fee you charge is too little, the common perception of students is that you are not very good. If you charge a lot, the common perception is that you are greedy.

My Sifu's grandfather was a master of Southern Boxing, who taught the youths in his village; he also ran the local opium den. He was paid for the tuition in rice and the fiery local alcohol. However, he strongly advised my Sifu not to teach hard-style martial arts because there was no money in it. Instead he said to him, 'Your uncle teaches Tai Chi Chuan; learn from him and you can meet wealthy merchants and officials who will pay you a lot of money to learn Tai Chi to improve their health.'

My teacher followed his grandfather's advice and began learning Tai Chi from his uncle. He found it very unsatisfactory as his uncle knew very little about the martial aspects and taught Tai Chi mainly for health purposes. The situation was remedied when his uncle heard from another instructor of a master, Qi Minxuan, from Henan province. In 1946 he invited Qi to Hong Kong to teach his sons and nephew. Qi taught Tai Chi as a fighting art. He taught the complete art to my Sifu,

receiving his bed and board in return. Qi didn't care about money. He was a devout Buddhist who had lost everything, including his family, in the war. In the winter of 1948, he left Hong Kong. My Sifu never saw him again.

Before leaving, Qi told my Sifu that recent generations of the well-known Tai Chi families had no interest in teaching the practical applications of the techniques.

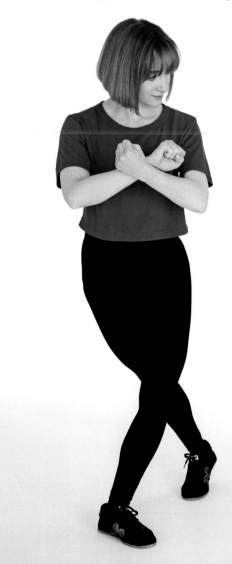

As a result, there were few practitioners of high quality and this made others despise Tai Chi Chuan. He told the teenage Cheng Tin-hung that, if he wished to teach and develop the art, he had to be sound in mind and body and able to defend himself properly; because of this Qi did not dare to keep anything secret from him.

At the age of 18, my Sifu became a full-time professional Tai Chi tutor. With many old and famous members of the well-known Tai Chi families teaching the art in Hong Kong, you might wonder who would go to a teenager. But people did.

Some of the old masters went to see my Sifu and remonstrate with him for teaching so many aspects of the art so openly. In particular, they were angry that he taught Neigong and other 'inside the door' training from a fairly early stage and over a short period of time, instead of waiting at least six years and even then teaching only a couple of techniques a year.

Until a few years ago there were very few people in Europe teaching Tai Chi weapons, self-defence and Neigong; Pushing Hands knowledge was limited. At that time some teachers did not give value for money. They did not actively cheat their students, but they taught very little and asked a lot.

One teacher of high repute always tantalized students with the prospect that one day they might be taught the Sword. That day never arrived. Another refused to teach the Sword on the grounds that it was too violent. Even those who do teach the Sword often don't teach applications.

I've been making a living out of Tai Chi since 1984. The main reason people seek me out as a Tai Chi tutor is that they want their Tai Chi to be empowered and don't want to waste their time. One thing that has struck me is the great humility exhibited by some of those I taught. Many of these students have been teaching martial arts for a long time and are professional instructors.

In turn they have taught me a great deal by telling me about their methods and experiences. Whenever possible I like to watch them teaching, so that I can learn ways of improving my own teaching technique. The Chinese call this type of student part student, part friend.

I have been learning Chinese on and off since 1975. My teachers have been from Hong Kong, Taiwan and mainland China. All had that most vital of requirements, a sense of humour.

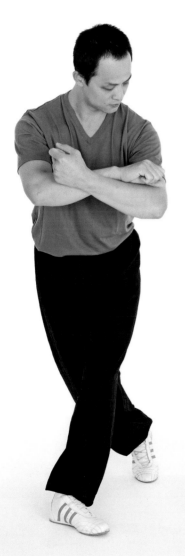

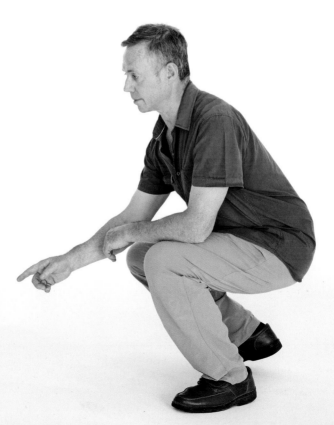

Certified Instructors

Over the last 25 years there have been and continue to be attempts by different Tai Chi and Chinese martial arts bodies in many countries to assess and categorize Tai Chi tutors. This is something of a reprise of the situation that prevailed in Japanese martial arts 40–50 years ago.

The Chinese authorities in China and Taiwan seek to control what they see as their birthright, while Westerners prefer non-interference. Here are some of the approaches used. I have chosen a few different examples for the purpose of comparison, but the list of bodies that certify Tai Chi and Qigong instructors given here is by no means exhaustive.

China

The Chinese Wushu (martial arts) authorities introduced nine Duan/levels to assess practitioners of Chinese martial arts, including Tai Chi. The first three levels are termed Beginner, the next three are Intermediate and the final three Advanced. It takes progressively longer for practitioners to achieve a higher level. It is also progressively more expensive.

The UK

The Tai Chi Union for Great Britain has opted for a simpler approach since its formation in 1991. Instructor members are divided into four instructor levels which are awarded by the Executive Committee:

Senior instructors (S) will normally have at least 20 years' experience of practising Chinese internal arts

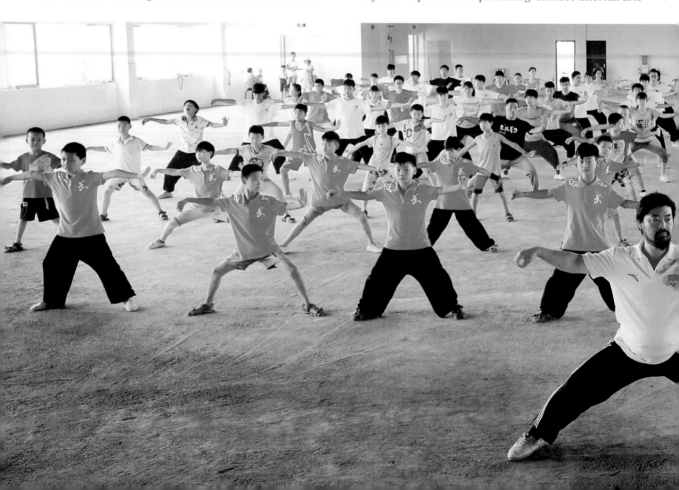

in depth; they may vote at General Meetings, stand for election to the Executive Committee (EC) and are in theory qualified to be members of the Technical Panel.

Advanced instructors (A) will normally have at least 8–10 years' experience of practising Chinese internal arts in depth; they may vote at General Meetings and stand for election to the EC.

Intermediate instructors (I) must be able to practise Chinese internal arts to an acceptable level; they may vote at General Meetings, but not stand for election to the EC.

Basic instructors (B) are continuing their apprenticeship in Chinese internal arts and are able to teach at a basic level; they may attend General Meetings but not vote or stand for election.

Control of the organization therefore rests in the hands of the most senior members.

France

In 2010, the French Wushu (martial arts) Federation published specific regulations for the awarding of Duan (levels) in Tai Chi; these include 'multiple and complementary approaches from the domains of health, energetics, martial arts and philosophy'.

More specifically the examiners look at balance, coordination, rooting, intent and other such important qualities, whether with or without weapons and whether doing forms or applications. The regulations are quite detailed and even specify the type of clothing to be worn by examinees.

Let's look at some examples. To obtain a First Duan, the candidate must show 3–5 minutes of basic exercises or 3–5 minutes of a form from a recognized style of Tai Chi, single- and double-hand Fixed Step Pushing Hands and five applications of form movements. For Second Duan, he is assessed doing five minutes of form or basic exercises, then he is required to show named techniques from the Hand Form and their application. He is also required to know the Eight Forces and their names in Chinese, as well as showing how to practise Fixed Step Pushing Hands.

The testing gets progressively stiffer up to Sixth Duan, at higher levels requiring a written thesis. Beyond Sixth Duan, awards are honorary.

Other European Countries

For more than 25 years there has been a highly effective Taijiquan and Qigong Network in Germany, essentially operating as a professional body looking after members' interests.

Below In China, the path to becoming a qualified practitioner takes longer to achieve the more advanced you become.

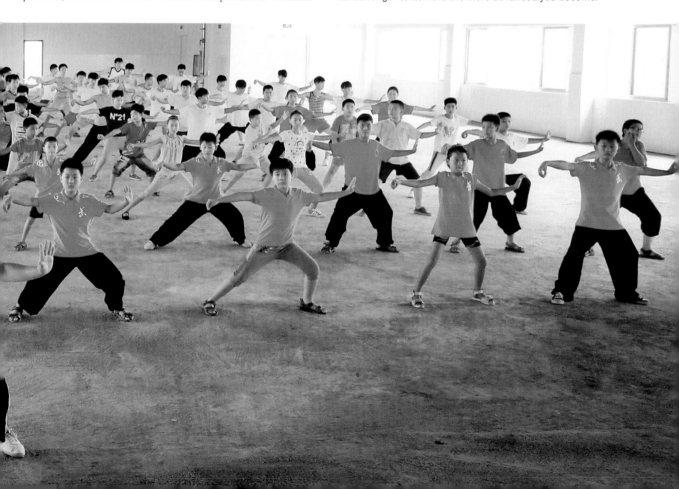

The Dutch had an effective Stichting/organization for years, but it relied mainly on one person who is much less involved now. They are in the process of restructuring.

There are loose structures in some of the Scandinavian countries, but no formal national Tai Chi organizations.

The Austrian Taijiquan and Qigong Association is a well-run national organization.

In Spain there are some major Tai Chi events and informal contact between groups, but no real structure.

Many national European organizations are members of the Taijiquan and Qigong Federation of Europe (TCFE), which organizes annual events, including competitions.

The USA

There is no national Tai Chi body in the USA, but there is a National Qigong Association. I was invited as a foreign guest instructor to their 2001 National Qigong Gathering ('Moving into wholeness; the transformational power of Qigong') by an old pal, Jim MacRitchie, who is also a Qigong author.

The programme said, 'The National Qigong (Chi Kung) Association (NQA) is the umbrella organization that embraces and supports equally all schools, traditions, teaching styles and philosophies of Qigong and Tai Chi. We are a professional organization as well as a community of Qigong enthusiasts with all levels of experience.' From my observations this is an accurate description of the NQA as evidenced by the presence of a group of Falun Gong practitioners.

The most interesting though technical lecture and seminar at the gathering was from Dr Lili Feng on 'Recent Discoveries in Scientific Qigong Research'.

What set the whole event apart from a proper academic approach to an art or science was that nobody seemed to want to question anything, no matter how bizarre or obscure; everything was indeed 'embraced and supported equally'. In one sense this is noble, in another it means that the Chinese internal arts have a credibility gap that cannot be narrowed until a more scientific approach is adopted.

I also attended an important panel presentation: 'Standards, Credentials and National Examinations in Clinical Qigong'. The panel discussed suggested requirements such as 'instructors' having a minimum of 200 hours tuition over two years including (most sensibly) a 'Qi Deviation Class'; while 'medical specialists' would be expected to have 400 hours of experience in Qigong and related subjects such as anatomy, including a clinical element, over four years. There was also a suggestion that acupuncturists should teach Qi cultivation. These are all issues that we will have to face in Britain and Europe eventually. The Americans are dealing with them now.

Practical Tai Chi Chuan International – Instructor Certification

Further details of the assessment and classification of tutors by my own organization and by the French Wushu Federation are in Appendix II (see page 238–9).

Categorizing Tai Chi tutors into levels is probably a good thing in the main. But there are some excellent instructors who have never been assessed and many who have been assessed to a high level, but who really aren't very good. On a personal note, I was given a certificate from my Sifu in 1984 after having trained intensively with him since 1975, but there is no level on it; I'm also a Senior Instructor in, and founding member of, the Tai Chi Union for Great Britain.

Left Ultimately, a good Tai Chi instructor depends on their individual knowledge and ability.

Tai Chi Tutors and Martial Virtue

The Chinese martial arts have a concept called Wu De/Martial Virtue, which is supposed to govern a practitioner's behaviour when a physical conflict occurs. It is a kind of oriental chivalric code.

Wu De is concerned with morality in action as well as morality in thought. Morality in action governs our dealings with others; morality in thought enables us to be harmoniously spontaneous in our actions and reactions instead of being governed by our emotions or thinking instead of acting. The aim is to attain the state of Wu Chi/ Without Limits or No Ultimate – which may be why this is the first Tai Chi Hand Form posture.

The five virtues representing morality in action are humility, sincerity, courtesy, righteousness and trust. The Chinese term for righteousness, Yi, is a particularly interesting character. Its upper component represents a sheep or goat, while the lower component is I or me. Sheep and goats were sacrificial victims, so the concept is 'I sacrifice myself for others' – righteousness.

The five virtues representing morality in thought are courage, patience, endurance, perseverance and will. Ren is the term for patience; the upper component of the character represents a sharp weapon, the lower part is the heart, so we have a wounded heart. By extension the meaning is to sustain or be patient.

In my experience martial virtue, like Tai Chi effectiveness, is easier in the theory than in the practice. My own Sifu was very far from being a paragon of either of these two sets of virtues, but he was sincere in his teachings. Always something of a chancer, in 1976 when I was representing Hong Kong at the Fourth Southeast Asian Championships in Singapore, he offered me anabolic steroids. I refused.

At the same competition, I won two gruelling fights to get into the final of the Heavyweight Division. My opponent was the Malaysian Heavyweight Boxing Champion. He'd been drawn against his own brother in the semi-final and the brother had withdrawn to give him a bye into the final. He was completely fresh and bigger and heavier than I was. I had two black eyes, a bleeding nose, cut lips, swelling and bruising from stamps and kicks all down my left side, so bad that I couldn't get my shoe on properly. I knew I'd lose. Sifu told me that I didn't have to fight; everyone would understand. I told him that I had to fight or people would say I was afraid. He beat me, of course, but not by much. I had to wait four years,

until the next Southeast Asian Championships, to come back to beat him in the final in Kuala Lumpur. In martial arts reputation is everything.

Just before this, the undisputed World Heavyweight Boxing Champion Muhammad Ali had fought a Japanese wrestler. One day I went to train with Sifu as usual, only to find his studio packed out with members of the Hong Kong press. He'd issued a press release that his student, Inspector Dan Docherty of the Royal Hong Kong Police Force, challenged Ali to a fight where he would use Tai Chi to defeat Western boxing. Faced with a fait accompli, I went along with it. Perhaps wisely, Ali did not reply.

Despite what I've said, I do believe in martial virtue. I've seen the way people change through martial arts. Since he was 11 years old, my son has trained with me in Tai Chi and has been my partner of choice when demonstrating techniques. He can be trusted to do techniques which demand control of bladed weapons. He has become self-disciplined and responsible. I can rely on him when he is training with beginners. He isn't the first youth to be changed by martial arts practise, nor will he be the last.

Tai Chi Tutors Talking

I've included here a variety of questions from Tai Chi tutors with varying amounts of experience.

Questions from Carol

Q: The concepts of Qi, Jing and Shen are clearly rooted in centuries of Eastern philosophy, and as such are difficult for Westerners to grasp fully, as we don't have the background ideas, history and nuances of language. While some students are happy to accept them in an almost mystical sense, others are not. How can these concepts be explained to those whose background lies in Western medical ideas and rational scientific/evidence-based thought?

My teacher took a practical view of these three concepts, and I do, too. Qi is more or less breath and circulation. Jing refers to the vital essences such as semen, sweat and saliva. Shen is the spirit or psyche. If there is anything wrong with any one of these Three Treasures, the other two will also be adversely affected (for more about the concept of the Three Treasures, see pages 80–1). One of the primary aims of Tai Chi practice is to maximize the amount of Qi taken into and used up by the body and thereby to stimulate the production of vital essences and of Shen.

Q: Many new students are attracted to Tai Chi because of the idea that it is gentle exercise and will help to improve balance and flexibility for injured joints. This can lead to students asking for advice that would perhaps be better given by qualified physiotherapists and other professionals who have spent years formally studying human anatomy and physiology, rather than a tutor for whom Tai Chi may be a part-time 'hobby'. How can you encourage injured students with reliable, safe, movements/drills while avoiding becoming open to claims of worsening their situation?

Firstly, anyone with an existing medical condition should inform their Tai Chi tutor so that the tutor can give appropriate tuition. It is advisable to seek out an experienced Tai Chi teacher, and not just go to the one who is nearest. Unfortunately it always comes back to finding a competent and experienced tutor who can explain correct principles.

Questions from Stephen

Q: I have noted that many instructors in a number of different arts use the term centre line. I would be interested to know how you describe this. Can you also explain why it is important for both defence and offence and how you teach the concept?

The nose is in the centre of the face, the spinal column is the exact centre of the body. When straight-punching an opponent, we want the body weight and therefore the spinal column to be behind the punch with the torso leaning forward, so that everything is going forward. This is spinal flexion. With spinal rotation we turn the centre line to generate greater force, in both attack and defence. Sometimes we generate spinal flexion and spinal rotation in the same technique. This is common in sports such as tennis and golf as well as martial arts.

Q: How are advanced practitioners able to withstand blows to their body? I understand that Neigong must be practised. However, I have seen you demonstrate the ability to take two flying kicks. At the point of impact, what are you doing to receive these blows? Are you relaxed, breathing in to your diaphragm, breathing out or perhaps bracing your body? You once said, 'Be like a sponge.' What does that mean?

People like to talk about 'iron shirt', but iron shirt isn't part of Tai Chi and essentially is a term imported from sagas about Chinese knights errant. To take the kicks you need to brace yourself and absorb rather than stiffen when you receive the impact.

Questions from Danny

Q: How do you maintain the balance of attention between loyal and ongoing students and new recruits? I always find this hard as new recruits demand more of my attention, but obviously come and go much more than the loyal and long term, who can easily be overlooked.

Beginners always need more attention. More experienced students can be asked to do some training with beginners to get them started. Another way is to have an extra half-hour or so for advanced students or arrange for small groups of advanced students to do some private training sessions with their tutor on a regular basis.

Q: How is it best to divide time between forms/ Qigong and Pushing Hands/applications? Most of my students are more drawn towards learning and practising forms rather than developing Pushing Hands skills and learning/improving applications – my hope is that students run through forms/Qigong in their own time and classes are spent on aspects that cannot be studied without partners to work with. Getting this balance right always seems to be a struggle.

There isn't much point in forcing people to do things that they don't want to do. Either they need to practise different things at the same time or the tutor needs to find some extra time for applications.

Q: How do you keep ongoing and old students – and teachers, come to that – motivated to move forward, and move them away from bad habits?

Experienced students need to be given the opportunity to practise more advanced skills. From time to time, it's also good to do a forms clinic. It's not enough for the tutor to say something is wrong; he needs to explain why that is so.

Q: How important is it to maintain the structure and detail of the system that you learn as opposed to developing your own style and approach?

Tai Chi is an art, so we all do it a bit differently. It becomes ours. The structure needs to be accurate, and we don't want to lose the detail. Everything that should be there must be there, but there are also permissible variations in tempo and technique which you gradually become aware of. Art isn't just about copying. It's about expressing the essence of what is there.

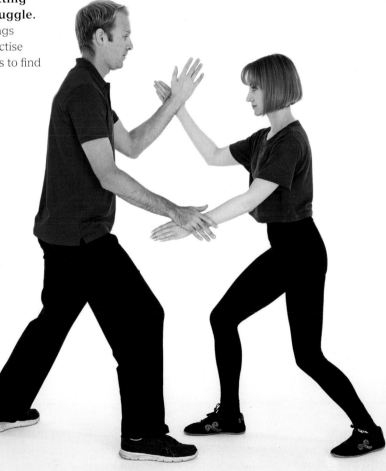

Glossary

13 tactics Old name for Tai Chi Chuan, referring to the Eight Forces/tactics and the Five Steps.

64 hexagrams Figures of Six broken and/or unbroken lines used for divination in *The Book of Changes*.

An A downward press. One of the Eight Forces/tactics.

Application training Practicing self-defence techniques with a partner.

Back stance Most of the weight is on the rear foot.

Bagua Eight trigrams which combine to make up the 64 hexagrams of *The Book of Changes*.

Baguazhang 8 Trigram Palm. Martial art based on Bagua.

Bian To change.

The Book of Changes (*Yi Jing/I Ching*) Book of divination dating back more than 3,000 years.

Cai To uproot. One of the Eight Forces/tactics.

Canon of Tai Chi Chuan One of the five major Tai Chi Chuan Classics.

Chen Tuan (906-899 CE) Taoist alchemist and philosopher.

Chuan The literal meaning is fist, so it has come to mean martial art as in Tai Chi Chuan.

The Classic of the Way and Virtue Taoist writings of Laozi (c. 4th century BCE)

Da Lu/Big Diversion Advanced Tai Chi pushing hands method. Also known as Four Corners and Eight Gates, Five Steps.

Dantian In internal alchemy there are three Dantrian; for Tai Chi purposes, we are only concerned with the Cinnabar Field just below the navel. Key point in internal alchemy.

Dao A Way/the Way or Ways.

Dao Sabre or broadsword.

Daoyin Leading and conducting energy flow.

Die Pu Fall hit. Making the opponent fall and then hitting him or hitting him to make him fall.

Dim Mak Attacking vital points.

Doctrine of the Mean/Zhong Yong One of the Confucian classics.

Double-weightedness Absence of Yin and Yang.

Duan Level/grade.

Eight Forces Peng, Lu, Ji, An, Cai, Lie, Zhou, Kao.

Exercise of The Five Animals/Five Animal Frolic Hygienic exercise attributed to the famous physician, Hua Tuo (3rd century BCE)

External alchemy/Wai Dan) Use of herbs/drugs etc. to stimulate the life force.

Fa Jin Discharging force.

Fighters Song One of the five major Tai Chi Chuan Classics.

Five Element Arm Tai Chi self defence drill.

Flying Flower Palm Tai Chi striking drill.

Form Including Long Form, Short Form, Round Form, Hand Form. Choreographed sequences of martial arts movements.

Four Emblems Old/Young Yin/Yang as represented by the four possible two lined variations of broken/unbroken lines.

Front stance Most of the weight is on the front foot.

Guoshu National Art/usually refers to Chinese full-contact fighting.

He Kai Closing and opening.

Heguanzi Heguanzi Pheasant Cap Master.

Hua Often translated as to transform/to change/to convert.

Hua jin Using skilled force to redirect the opponent's force.

Hun Tun (Chaos) which is also Tai Chi (Supreme/Ultimate Pole).

Internal Alchemy Working on the Three Treasures, Qi, Jing, Shen.

Internal Family Boxing Mainly refers to Tai Chi Chuan, Baguazhang and Xingyi.

Ji Push/diverse force. One of Tai Chi's Eight Forces.

Jia Family. Can refer to martial arts.

Jian Straight Sword.

Jibengong Basic skills.

Jin Skilled force.

Jingshen Vigour/vital essences and spirit.

Jingzuo Quiet sitting meditation.

Kao To lean/barge. One of Tai Chi's forces/tactics.

Laozi 'The Old Boy'; Chinese philosopher (c. 4th century BCE).

Lei Tai Platform for Chinese full-contact fighting.

Li Strength.

Lie Spiralling. One of the Eight Forces/tactics.

Lineages Martial art lines of transmission.

Lu Sideways diversion. One of Tai Chi's Eight Forces/tactics.

Men Gate/door. Metaphor for a martial arts style.

Mencius Leading Confucian (4th century BCE).

Mian Cotton / soft.

Nei Dan Internal Alchemy.

Neigong Internal strength training.

Pai School / style.

Peng Upward force. One of Tai Chi's Eight Forces/tactics.

Pushing hands/Tui Shou Methods of partner training at close distance.

Qi Vital energy.

Qiang Spear.

Qigong Training vital energy circulation.

Qin Na Seizing and holding.

Reeling Silk Pushing hands method in Wu lineage / Body concept of Chen style.

Running Thunder Hand Tai Chi fighting drill.

San Shou Literally means scattering hands; fighting techniques.

Seven Stars Reference to the Great Bear / Northern Dipper.

Shen Spirit.

Shi Technique.

Shuai Jiao Chinese wrestling.

Sifu Literally means teaching father.

Six Harmonies and Eight Methods Chinese internal martial art.

Shaolin Name of a series of Chan Buddhist temples where martial arts were practised.

Sui Following. Tai Chi strategy.

Suspended headtop Correct alignment of head and spine.

Tai Chi Concept of Supreme Pole/Ultimate.

Tao/dao Sabre/broadsword.

Wai Dan External alchemy.

Wu Chi No Ultimate.

Wu De Martial virtue.

Wushu Martial arts.

Wu Wei Taoist concept of non-action.

Wu Xing Five Elements.

Xin Heart mind.

Yang The active/male principle.

Yi Intent.

Yin The passive / female principle.

Zhongzheng Centrally correct.

Zhou Forearm. One of the Eight Forces/tactics.

Zhou Dunyi (1017–73 CE) Neo-Confucian.

Zhuangzi Taoist philosopher (c. 5th century BCE).

Zhu Xi (1130-1200 CE) Neo-Confucian.

Zou To move (the feet).

APPENDIX I:
Tai Chi Techniques Name Comparisons

The Classic of Boxing lists 32 techniques taken from 16 schools of boxing – Tai Chi wasn't one of them. Of those 32 techniques 29 are found in Chen lineage and 8 of the techniques are found in Yang lineage. This means that all Chen and Yang lineage schools are practicing non-Tai Chi techniques.

About 22 Chen Tai Chi form techniques have the same or a similar name to those of Yang lineage Long Form and around 26 of the techniques have names which are wholly or partly different from Yang Long Form techniques. Around 11 techniques from the Chen Pao Chui form have the same or a similar name to those of Yang lineage Long Form and around 33 of the techniques have names which are wholly or partly different from Yang Long Form techniques. (There are many variations in both original Chinese lists and in different translated versions of many of the terms.)

In the Wu lineage Long Form (see page 235), which has more variation than classical Yang style, there are 23 techniques with different names from Chen style form techniques.

My conclusion is that *The Classic of Boxing* influenced both Chen style and Tai Chi Chuan to different degrees, and later, after Yang Luchan made Tai Chi famous, the Chens absorbed it into their system.

Techniques featured in *The Classic of Boxing* and in the Yang Lineage

The column on the right lists the eight techniques which are also found in Yang style.

Number	Classic of Boxing	Yang
1.	Lazy Tying a Coat	Grasping Bird's Tail (sounds similar to Lazy Tying a Coat)
2.	Golden Cockerel on One Leg	Golden Cockerel on One Leg
3.	Pat the Horse	Pat the Horse High
4.	Bent Single Whip	Single Whip
5.	Seven Star Fists	Seven Stars
6.	Reverse Ride Dragon	-
7.	Two Changes of the Legs	-
8.	Qiu and Liu Technique	-
9.	Low Insert Technique	-
10.	Lie in Ambush Technique	(looks similar to Draw the Bow to Shoot the Tiger)
11.	Throw Technique	-
12.	Lift Forearm Technique	-
13.	With Sudden Steps Respond Rapidly	-
14.	Seize and Hold Technique	-
15.	Centralize Four Levels	-
16.	Crouching Tiger Technique	-
17.	High Four Levels Body Method	-
18.	Invert and Insert Technique	-
19.	Well Fence Four Levels	-
20.	Demon Kicks	-
21.	Point at Groin	Punch the Groin
22.	Beast Head	-
23.	Spirit Fist	-
24.	One Whip	-
25.	Sparrow Earth Dragon	-
26.	Facing Sun Hand	-
27.	Wild Goose Wings	-
28.	Ride Tiger	Step Back to Ride Tiger
29.	Twist Arms like the Luan	-
30.	Aim at Head Cannon	-
31.	Smoothly Use Luan Zhou	-
32.	Flag and Drum Technique	-

Chen Lineage Tai Chi Form Techniques

Techniques which are also found in Yang style are highlighted in **bold**. Some names are partially in bold as they are partially the same.

1. **Preparing Form**
2. Buddha's Warrior Attendant Pounds Mortar
3. **Lazy About Tying Coat**
4. Six Sealing and Four Closing
5. **Single Whip**
6. **The White Crane Spreads Its Wings**
7. Walk Obliquely and **Twist Step** on Both Sides
8. The First Closing
9. Wade Forward and Twist Step on Both Sides
10. The Second Closing
11. The Fist of Covering Hand and Arm
12. The Punch of **Draping Over the Body**
13. Lean With Back
14. The Blue Dragon Goes Out of Water
15. Push Both Hands
16. Change Palms Three Times
17. **The Punch at Elbow's Bottom**
18. Step Back and Whirl Arms on Both Sides
19. Step Back and Press Elbow
20. Middle Winding
21. **Flash the Back**
22. **Cloud Hands**
23. **High Pat on Horse**
24. **Rub with Right and Left Foot**
25. **Kick with Left and Right Heel**
26. **The Punch of Hitting the Ground**
27. Turn Over Body and Double-Raise Foot
28. Beast's Head Pose
29. Tornado Foot
30. Small Catching And Hitting
31. Forward Trick
32. Backward Trick
33. **Part the Wild Horse's Mane on Both Sides**
34. Shake Both Feet
35. **The Jade Girl Works at Shuttles**
36. Shake Foot and Stretch Down
37. **Golden Cockerel Stands on One Leg**
38. **Cross Waving Lotus**
39. **The Punch of Hitting Crotch**
40. The White Ape Presents Fruit
41. The Dragon on the Ground
42. **Step Forward with Seven Stars**
43. **Step Back and Mount the Tiger**
44. **Turn Body and Double Wave Lotus**
45. The Cannon Right Overhead
46. **Closing Form**

Chen Lineage Pao Chui Form Techniques

Techniques which are also found in Yang style are highlighted in **bold**. Some names are partially in bold as they are partially the same.

1. **Preparing Form**
2. Buddha's Warrior Attendant Pounds Mortar
3. **Lazy About Tying Coat**
4. Six Sealing and Four Closing
5. **Single Whip**
6. Move and Hinder with Elbow (in Yang lineage this is Deflect Parry and Punch)
7. The Fist of Protecting Heart
8. **Twist Step on Both Sides** and Walk Obliquely
9. Sink Waist with Elbow Down
10. Go Straight with Left Palm into Well
11. Plum Blossoms Scattered by the Wind
12. The Fist of Protecting Body
13. The Fist of Putting Fists aside before Body
14. Cut Hand
15. Turn Flowers out and Brandish Sleeves
16. The Fist of Covering Hand and Arm
17. Jump a Step and Twist Elbow
18. **Cloud Hands**
19. **Pat High on Horse**
20. Cannons in Series
21. Ride the Animal in the Reverse Direction
22. **The White Snake Spits its Tongue**
23. Turn Flowers out from **the Bottom of the Sea**
24. Turn Body with Six Closings
25. Wrap Crackers

26. Beast's Head Pose
27. Splitting Pose
28. Tame the Tiger
29. The Hitting of Rubbing Eyebrow Makes Red
30. The Yellow Dragon Stirs Water Three Times
31. **Kick with Left and Right Heel**
32. Sweeping Leg
33. Dash Leftward and Rightward
34. Thrust Reversely

35. Attack Twice with Forearm
36. Linking Cannons
37. **The Jade Girl Works at Shuttles**
38. The Cannon of Turning Head
39. Smooth Elbows
40. The Elbow of Hitting Heart
41. The Cannon out of Bosom
42. **Closing Form**

Wu Lineage Tai Chi Form Techniques

Techniques which are not found in Chen style are highlighted in **bold**. I have given one asterisk (*) to techniques which have an equivalent in Chen lineage under a different name and two asterisks (**) where a similar move is found in Chen style but there is no name for it in Chen.

1. Beginning Style* (includes Tai Chi at Rest/Wu Chi and Ready Position/Tai Chi)
2. **Vanguard Arms**
3. **Extend Arms**
4. **Seven Stars Style**
5. Grasping Bird's Tail*
6. **Single Whip**
7. **Flying Oblique High and Low**
8. **Single Hand Seize Legs**
9. **Double Hands Seize Legs**
10. **Raise Hands and Step Up**
11. White Crane Flaps its Wings
12. **Break-arm Style**
13. Brush Knee Twist Step*
14. **Stroke the Lute**
15. Deflect, Parry and Punch* (includes inner form technique Use the Forearm to Force the Door)
16. **As if Shutting a Door**
17. **Embrace Tiger, Return to Mountain**
18. **Cross Hands**
19. Fist under Elbow
20. Step Back Repulse Monkey
21. Needle at Sea Bottom

22. Fan through the Back
23. **Swing Fist**
24. Cloud Hands
25. Pat the Horse High
26. **Separate Hands**
27. Tiger Embraces Head**
28. Drape Body Left and Right*
29. Separate Feet Left and Right*
30. Turn Body and Kick with Heel
31. Step Forward Plant the Punch*
32. **Turn Body and Swing Fist**
33. **Step Back Seven Stars**
34. **Beat the Tiger**
35. **Drape Body and Kick** (also known as Two Raisings of the Foot)
36. **Box the Ears**
37. Parting Wild Horse's Mane
38. Fair Lady Works Shuttle
39. **Snake Creeps Down (low style)**
40. Golden Cockerel Stands on One Leg
41. White Snake Spits out Tongue
42. **Slap the Face**
43. Single Hand Sweep Lotus Leg
44. Punch the Groin
45. Step Up Seven Stars
46. Step Back to Ride the Tiger
47. Double Hand Sweep Lotus Leg
48. **Draw the Bow to Shoot the Tiger***
49. **Tai Chi in Unity and Completion Style**

APPENDIX II:
Instructor Assessment Requirements

USA National Qigong Association Instructor Certification Requirements

Qigong Teacher Track

Level I Qigong Instructor: This is the initial level for an instructor of Qigong. It requires at least 200 hours of documented formal Qigong training.

Level II Qigong Instructor: At this level the instructor gives instruction in technical forms and tries to improve their students' quality of life. It requires at least 350 hours of documented formal Qigong training.

Level III Advanced Instructor: The Advanced Instructor has a higher level of understanding of the practice as well as its benefits. Advanced Instructors should be able to generate Qi, absorb Qi from the atmosphere, and have trained their Qi (how all this can be measured, I do not know). They have built a strong energetic foundation through disciplined practice of Qigong and possess an understanding of healing principles. This requires at least 500 hours of documented formal Qigong training and at least five years of Qigong teaching experience.

Level IV Teacher: This is the top level of recognition. Level IV practitioners have taught instructors of Qigong or Qigong clinical therapists for ten years or more. They act as mentors for others in the field and are acknowledged senior practitioners by the NQA. This level is recognized to teach all levels of formal instruction.

At least 1,000 hours of documented formal instruction in Qigong, at least ten years of Qigong teaching and the passing of an interview process are required. These interviews are held by at least three members of the Application Review Committee.

A student of a Level IV NQA Certified Teacher may supply a strong letter of recommendation from the teacher that includes the number of hours of relevant instruction, general description of coursework and descriptive comments about student ability, instead of listing course information from that teacher in his or her application.

Clinical Track

Clinical Practitioner: This title is given to those who practise healing Qigong with emission and projection of Qi and may also teach prescriptive exercises. People at this level have the ability to generate Qi, absorb Qi from the atmosphere, and have trained their Qi. They have built a strong energetic foundation through practice of Qigong and understand healing principles. This requires at least 500 hours of documented formal Qigong training, including at least 350 didactic hours, 200 of which are specific to Qigong, and at least 100 hours of Qigong treatment. This may include contact and non-contact Qi emission, adjunct massage manipulations, teaching of prescriptive exercises or any combination thereof. The Clinical Practitioner must also have at least two years' clinical experience and must carry a current liability insurance policy.

Advanced Clinical Therapist: This level is set to mentor and teach others in the art, science and skills necessary for Qigong healing/medical Qigong. This requires at least 1,500 hours of documented formal Qigong training, including at least 500 didactic hours, 350 of which are specific to Qigong, and at least 1,000 hours of Qigong treatment. The Advanced Clinical Therapist must also have at least ten years' clinical experience and must carry a current liability insurance policy.

A person may hold certification as both Teacher and Clinical Practitioner: this is referred to below as an 'add on'. Members will receive a certification listing on their member page of the NQA website, a resource for those seeking a professional with distinction. NQA publications may regularly highlight certified professionals with articles about them and their practice.

Initial certification (from $150) extends for two years, except for Level IV Teacher, which has a higher fee due to the needed interview. Renewals are anywhere from $50 and extend for two years. An upgrade or add-on is from $100 except for the Level IV Teacher, which will be more.

A continuing education requirement for renewal may be initiated at some point in the future.

A didactic hour of instruction is received in a class setting from an instructor rather than clinical practice with patients.

You may submit an upgrade by entering the additional information on a new application and send it in along with the appropriate fee.

Practical Tai Chi Chuan International Nine-Level Teacher Certification System

This is the organization that I set up in 1984. Its nine levels are:

Level 1	Jing	Essence	Junior Instructor
Level 2	Ming	Comprehension	Assistant Instructor
Level 3	Zhi	Judicious	Basic Level Instructor
Level 4	Hui	Vitality	Intermediate Instructor
Level 5	Qian	Humility	Senior Instructor
Level 6	Xu	Void	Advanced Instructor
Level 7	Ren	Fortitude	Master
Level 8	Rang	Oral	Chief Instructor
Level 9	Yu	The Fool	Principal Instructor

Criteria for Instructor Certificates

The following is a general guide only, and any level can be influenced by other factors.

Level 1: Basic postures and stances done correctly + some knowledge of Tui Shou.

Level 2: Short Form (square and round) + basic Tui Shou Fixed and Moving Step.

Level 3: Long Form + most Tui Shou Fixed and Moving Step + Basic San Shou applications + Basic Qigong (Cloud Hands, Tiger Embracing Head, Retrieving Moon from Sea, Single Hand Sweeps Lotus Leg) + one weapon.

Level 4: Long Form (square and round) + one weapon + Bai Shi + major San Shou techniques.

Level 5: Advanced Short Form + two weapons + Da Lu + two-person set (Sabre and Sabre/Staff) + philosophy/theory + conditioning exercises + 12 Yin Neigong.

Level 6: Three weapons + 12 Yang Neigong or Xian Jia Baduanjin Qigong + most San Shou techniques + mirror Short and Long Form + two mirror weapons forms.

Level 7: Xian Jia Baduanjin Qigong + 12 Yang Neigong + all 48 San Shou techniques (including variations) + Eight Forces for each weapon + Zhou Lu + three mirror weapons forms.

Level 8: Cai Lang + Six Secret Words + Fei Hua Zhang + reverse Long Form + full weapons applications + additional influencing factors.

Level 9: All aspects of Wudang Tai Chi Chuan + many additional influencing factors.

Additional influencing factors
In addition to the above, any level can be influenced by:

• Good attitude; entering/judging/refereeing Tai Chi competitions; attendance record at classes/seminars/workshops/camps; teaching classes; organizing events, etc.

• Seminars/workshops/demonstrations/camps; serving on national Tai Chi organisation committees; creating good publicity for Tai Chi; contribution to the Tai Chi community; visiting China and broadening your own and other people's general knowledge about the development and benefits of Tai Chi, writing Tai Chi related articles/reviews, etc.

The French Wushu Federation – Chinese Energetic and Martial Arts

Tai Chi Chuan Duan Levels – Specific Regulations

Tai Chi Chuan belongs to Nei Jia (Chinese Internal Martial Arts).

Evaluation criteria

Chinese Internal Martial Arts are characterized by the existence of energetic and martial principles and the changes and harmonization of Yin and Yang. They are evaluated using multiple complementary approaches including health, energetics, martial arts and philosophy.

Specific criteria include:

1. Attitude and general presentation
2. Relaxation/release
3. Balance
4. Rooting
5. Staying in place, maintenance, stretching
6. Bows and structure
7. Connect upper/lower
8. Size and basin
9. Quality of shifting of weight
10. Quality of movements: intention, readability, density, fluidity, internal energy
11. Coordination
12. Quality of respiration
13. State: calm, concentrated and focused

Similar evaluation criteria exist for Neijia Wushu weapons.

Martial applications (Gong Fang)

1. Adaptability
2. Efficacy
3. Readability
4. Realism
5. Fluidity
6. Respect for partner

Pushing hands (Tui Shou)

1. Criteria as for Neijia Wushu sequences mentioned above
2. Criteria as for martial applications mentioned above
3. Contact with partner: absorption, ability to divert, adherence, discharging, direction

Outfits

Candidates must present themselves with their weapons and Chinese outfit or with the outfit of their school (long sleeves and pants) and suitable footwear.

They must provide a partner for martial applications and Pushing Hands.

Tai Chi Book Group

It's the information age – supposedly. There is a lot of information on Tai Chi available, but most of it is inaccurate. I don't take part in Internet discussion groups, but prefer to let my teaching and writings do the talking.

As we've seen, Tai Chi and the matters which touch upon it are complex and it's impossible to cover everything in depth in one book. People are interested in different things and, left to their own devices, don't always know where to go for further reading. So here's my answer to that, a list of books that are worth reading and discussing; recondite material not easily found in your local bookstores that addresses a wide variety of topics.

The Illustrated Canon of Chen Family Taijiquan

by Chen Xin; additional material by Chen Pan-ling;
translation by Alex Golstein
(INBI Matrix Property Ltd, 2007)

This seminal book on Chen style has assumed almost legendary status in some circles. Yet controversy dogged it before it was even written.

Tai Chi historian Wu Tunan (1884–1989) wrote of how he visited Chen Village in 1917 and met Chen Xin (1849–1929), who was a schoolmaster. Chen Xin announced he was working on a book connecting Tai Chi Chuan and the *Yi Jing*. According to Wu, Chen Xin told him that the Chen style of boxing was Pao Chui from the Shaolin Temple and that Tai Chi had been introduced to the village by Jiang Fa. Chen Xin also admitted he did not practise either Pao Chui or Tai Chi. Wu watched villagers practise under a teacher called Du Yuwan and observed that their Tai Chi was identical to that practised by the Yang family.

The Chen family claim that Chen Xin learned and taught their boxing, and wrote a Tai Chi guide for beginners. They are furious with Wu Tunan.

Senior Nationalist official, engineer and cult member Chen Pan-ling finished the book on Chen Xin's behalf. Left-wing Chinese martial arts historian Tang Hao arranged for it to be published.

More than 200 pages are devoted to *Yi Jing*, metaphysics, acupoints, internal alchemy, Tai Chi Chuan songs and 'classics'.

There is much discussion of silk reeling throughout the book, aligning it with acupoints and claiming it is impossible to practise Tai Chi without it. While the book includes some great Tai Chi from the other lineages, most of it is pretty poor stuff, with almost no body or limb torque being used during practice; it's to the Chens' credit that they emphasize the use of torque. You need a good structure.

The book also covers practical combat concepts such as attacking acupoints. It discusses applying specific techniques to specific acupoints in accordance with specific two-hour time periods; dubious indeed. There is no mention of silent contemplation to increase awareness, nor of consideration, deliberation or combining meditation and movement to achieve Qi control; these are qualities not always associated with Chen stylists. I do agree with the statement on visualization, 'Meditate on this move (Brush Knee Twist Step) and improvement will occur.' I also like the statement, 'Lack of beauty in Taiji practice cannot lead to mastery.'

Except for a short excerpt from *The Fighter's Song*, The Tai Chi Chuan Classics are not part of Chen style, but the book covers them in some detail. This is likely to be the work of Chen Pan-ling or Tang Hao, who would both be well acquainted with them.

The form is divided into 13 unequal sections of techniques, each section being efficacious physically, in terms of internal alchemy or as physical metaphors for philosophical concepts. This division of the form seems unique to the Chens.

There are two curious diagrams of boxers showing Wu Chi/No Ultimate or At Rest and Tai Chi/Supreme Ultimate. The Wu Chi model has a full head of hair; the Tai Chi chap is bald with a prominent crotch bulge. Strange?

The final and largest part of the book is a detailed discussion of all the techniques of the form in sequence, starting with Buddha's Warrior Attendant Pounding Mortar. Most Tai Chi practitioners are unaware that this technique occurs in a Shaolin form attributed to the first Song emperor, Taizu (960–76 CE).

The diagram of the technique comes with 17 pieces of advice. We are advised that orientation is not important, but then are told to face north, as this is the location of the Big Dipper (Ursa Major), 'the source of inherent energy in the human body'. We continue with an interesting diagram showing Qi flow through the body, which may well be based on a meditation posture of the Taoist Embrace the One meditative sect. This is followed by discussions on silk reeling and acupoints.

The author reveals how, when a callow youth, he suddenly realized that the entire mechanism of the technique Strike Down like Planting into the Ground depended on the concentration of Jing essence at the top of the head. It's hard to keep a straight face.

On the credit side, the book has some genuine points to make on Tai Chi practice. It is interesting as a historical document on Chen Tai Chi in pre-World War II years. It raises issues such as acupoints and internal alchemy which are rarely debated in a rational way by Tai Chi practitioners; and it is a valiant effort to present a huge array of difficult material, including many unusual diagrams. For those interested in Tai Chi Chuan history, it is essential reading.

Wu Style Tai Chi Chuan

by Wu Kung Cho
(Grand Master, 2006)

Wu Kung Cho was the elder son of Wu Jianquan and so was the senior member of the third generation of Wu family Tai Chi. In 1935, he published a book entitled *Wu Family Tai Chi Chuan*. In 1980, on being released from more than 20 years' penal servitude, he produced an edited version of the same book.

This new English-language edition is a far cry from the two Chinese versions; it presents the original texts and photos with new material in such a way as to make it a panegyric to the talents and accomplishments of family Wu. Such a eulogy may be justified given the part the Wu family has played in spreading Tai Chi – Wu lineage is second only to Yang in worldwide popularity. In terms of presentation the new book certainly outshines its predecessors, though many aspects of Wu-style Tai Chi such as the Nei Kung and specific Tui Shou sets are not discussed.

Wu Kung Cho introduces Zhang Sanfeng as Tai Chi's founder. He then mentions his grandfather's training under Yang Luchan before going on to explain key Tai Chi principles and specifically claiming Tai Chi to be a Taoist art. In the ninth of the Ten Essential Guidelines he mentions Tai Chi's highest achievement as being 'Plucking a Flower from the Wave's Crest'. The original Chinese text has Cai Lang Hua – literally 'Uprooting Wave Flower'. The third character is wrong and should be Hua, meaning to divert, so it should read 'Uprooting the Wave Diversion'. A solecism. A concept of Cai Lang Hua with different characters and meaning also exists in Chen style.

Wu later talks of 'Essentials of Winding Silk Jin'; his somewhat unclear explanation has the concept used in response to the opponent's actions. There is a Tui Shou drill and self-defence counters with the concept of reeling silk, which may be what he is referring to.

The most interesting part of the book is a collection of 40 texts said to have been given as a handwritten copy from Yang Banhou to Wu Quanyou. This would date these texts at sometime before 1892, when Yang died. The texts contain a mixture of Tai Chi theory, internal alchemy practice with sex as a metaphor for combat, details of Dim Mak (attacking pressure points) and a list of names of Tai Chi techniques which are no longer in use.

We can also compare photos of Wu Jianquan and his other son Wu Kungyi doing form techniques. The son looks a pale reflection of the father, though he was a hero for his 1954 brief encounter with the much younger White Crane stylist, Chan Hak Fu, whom I met many years later.

It is a flawed but fascinating book, of interest to the serious tutor and experienced practitioner. The Wu family like to play the role of Tai Chi custodians; in that case they owe us a bit more explanation. Sifu Eddie Wu, over to you.

Scholar Boxer

by Marnix Wells
(North Atlantic Books, 2005)

This book is about 'Chang Naizhou's Theory of Internal Martial Arts and the Evolution of Taijiquan'. Chang (1724–83) was a teacher of eclectic boxing and I've dealt with him earlier in the book as a historical snapshot (see page 58). At the time, under Emperor Qianlong, martial arts practice was proscribed and books about it were burned, so Chang's writings could circulate only among disciples. They were not published openly until after the 1911 revolution. However, there is some doubt about how much interpolation and extrapolation has been done to the text by persons other than Chang.

Marnix correctly identifies the many similarities between Chang's art and *The Classic of Boxing* and also Tai Chi Chuan. However, the differences are striking. In a great many of Chang's illustrations the centre line between the crown of the head and the coccyx is broken, with the head tilted up or down and the shoulders raised – all major structural defects in Tai Chi. There are many Buddhist references in the text, which suggest influences from the nearby Shaolin Temple. There are also Taoist and Confucian influences.

I asked Marnix how he felt Chang's art fitted into the scheme of things, in that Chang was based geographically between the Shaolin Temple and the Chen Village. He said it was hard to give the art a label because it is doubtful if anything is purely internal or external.

This is a difficult book that raises more questions than it answers. Marnix has done a considerable service to the Tai Chi community in writing it, though it is very much from a Chen-style perspective. It is, however, a must-read for the serious Tai Chi Chuan practitioner. As it says on the back cover, *Scholar Boxer* gives us as a rare insight into the practices of a bygone age at a time when the Manchu Qing Empire was at its peak.

Chen Pan-ling's Original Tai Chi Chuan Textbook

(Blitz, 1998)

Chen Pan-ling (1891–1967) is another mysterious Chinese internal martial artist known to us through the writings of Robert W Smith, who refers to him, in the foreword, as 'perhaps the most knowledgeable person in the world on the principles, rationale and practice of Chinese boxing at the time of his death'.

Chen was radical in his approach. He refused to Bai Shi, he was selective about whom he taught and he didn't charge. His Tai Chi teachers were Wu Jianquan, Yang Shaohou, Xu Yushen and Chi De. He also trained in the Chen family village, though we are not told with whom.

Chen developed his own idiosyncratic Tai Chi form with elements of Yang, Wu, Woo and Chen style in it, but it isn't widely practised outside Taiwan. I know of only one person in Britain practising Chen Pan-ling's Tai Chi.

In the historical section Chen adopts the conventional Chinese approach to religion of believing all truths, accepting the legitimacy of Chen Wangting, Zhang Sanfeng and the rest of the gang. A historian he was not.

Chen claims that his book contains the most elegant postures and most effective fighting techniques from the Yang, Chen and two Wu styles, yet no fighting technique is shown. He talks of a concept in advanced Tai Chi Chuan similar to radar, enabling masters to detect a surprise attack and to use invisible force to thrust the attacker away and to pick him up. A fighter Chen was not.

Chen is both interesting and informative in his discussions of breathing, movement, posture and the health benefits of form practice. Many of the layouts and charts, such as Chen's 20 Essential Points for Tai Chi Chuan, are effective ways of communicating his ideas to the reader, and his training as an engineer is evident in the methodical structure.

The conclusion I came to is that Chen Pan-ling had a lot of theoretical knowledge, but was weak on the practical level of how to use Tai Chi as a martial art, though he may have been a competent martial artist in other systems. The book contains a treasure trove of well-presented information that is likely to be of interest to novices and teachers of any Tai Chi school.

Martial Musings: A Portrayal of Martial Arts in the 20th Century
by Robert W Smith
(Via Media Publishing, 1999)

As we've seen (see page 65), Robert W Smith had a desk job with the CIA in Taiwan from 1959 to 1962. While there he met a bunch of people who were or subsequently became big names in Chinese martial arts and his reminiscences of these times are the best part of this book.

For Smith, a good teacher 'will be gentle, not forceful; he will be mild not blatant; he will be moderate and modest, but courageous'. Out of thousands of students, Smith gave permission to teach to only 12 who had spent more than five years with him.

The late Rose Li, a well-respected UK-based Tai Chi instructor and long-term pal of Smith, is given some typically constructive criticism, Smith concluding that her form is 'often double-weighted and not relaxed…the result of inadequate learning or dilution of Liu's original form by a young woman…' There is nothing about the opening up of mainland China and martial arts there, no history except recent history. Despite all this, the book is often interesting, with a wealth of opinions on people and styles from a time long gone.

For anyone interested in the passage of knowledge in the martial arts from Taiwan to the West, this book is indispensable.

The Harvard Medical School Guide to Tai Chi – 12 weeks to a Healthy Body, Strong Heart and Sharp Mind
by Peter M Wayne
(Shambhala Publications, 2013)

Dr Wayne is an Assistant Professor of Medicine and Director of Research at the world-renowned Harvard Medical School. His book is well written and unpretentious. Although a number of his quotes are incorrectly attributed to The Tai Chi Chuan Classics, I applaud his clear presentation of medical and scientific research based around the effectiveness of Tai Chi practice on a wide variety of medical conditions.

Dr Wayne has come up with 'Eight Active Ingredients of Tai Chi'. These are:

- Awareness
- Intention
- Structural integration
- Active relaxation
- Strengthening and flexibility
- Natural freer breathing
- Social support
- Embodies spirituality

These eight ingredients can be a useful way of looking at our Tai Chi practice and honing it to help alleviate a whole range of conditions.

Instead of teaching a traditional form, Dr Wayne has devised a purpose-built beginners' programme. He makes some perceptive remarks, pointing out that one of the attractions of Tai Chi is that it can enable students to be proactive in maintaining their health.

Tai Chi tutors will find the medical research and analysis of great value.

The Groves of Academe

The last 60 years or so have seen the growth of a Western academic approach to Tai Chi. In some respects this has been helpful. For example, the comparison tables of form names in Appendix I make the history of the origins of Tai Chi much clearer.

However, many of the Tai Chi writings translated over that period are problematic.

For example, in *Tai Chi Secret Transmissions*, translated by Professor Douglas Wile and published in 1983, Yang Chengfu is quoted as saying that the breathing should be in through the nose and out through the mouth, instead of out through the nose.

In another secret transmission a conversation is recorded between Yang Chengfu and his grandfather, Yang Luchan, though the grandfather had died before the grandson was born.

Why the lies?

Many of the applications shown by Yang Chengfu are absurd. Techniques are applied without footwork as they appear in the form. None of this is the fault of Professor Wile. Remember, we are in the world of truth and lies. Mao Zedong once said, 'No investigation, no right to speak.' A great many academics, armchair warriors and teenage scribbler Internet nerds would do well to remember that.

Further Reading

The insatiable Tai Chi bookworm may require further reading. The following writers are recommended:

Joseph Needham – on physiological alchemy. Although I previously mentioned that I find Needham too abstract, he does present wonderful material that it is not easy to find elsewhere in English.

Douglas Wile – translations of key Tai Chi writings.

Catherine Despeux – on Tai Chi and Daoyin.

David Palmer – on Qigong.

Livia Kohn/Kristoph Schipper – on internal alchemy.

The following studies may also be of interest:

Robinet, I. (1990) 'The Place and Meaning of the Notion of Taiji in Taoist Sources Prior to the Ming Dynasty', *History of Religions*, Vol. 29, No. 4, pp. 373–405
This is hard-core academia looking at the concept of Tai Chi and internal alchemy.

Ryan, A. (2009) 'Globalization and the "Internal Alchemy" in Chinese Martial Arts: the Transmission of Taijiquan to Britain', *East Asian Science, Technology and Society*, Vol. 2, No. 4, pp. 525–543
More of a social science approach to Tai Chi, but including a few decent stories.

Seidel, A. (1970) 'A Taoist Immortal of the Ming Dynasty: Chang San-feng' in De Bary, W T, *Self and Society in Ming Thought* (New York: Columbia University Press)
A most thorough and interesting study on the enigmatic Tai Chi patriarch.

APPENDIX IV:
Tai Chi Lineage Charts

Chart 1: Direct Chen family lineage

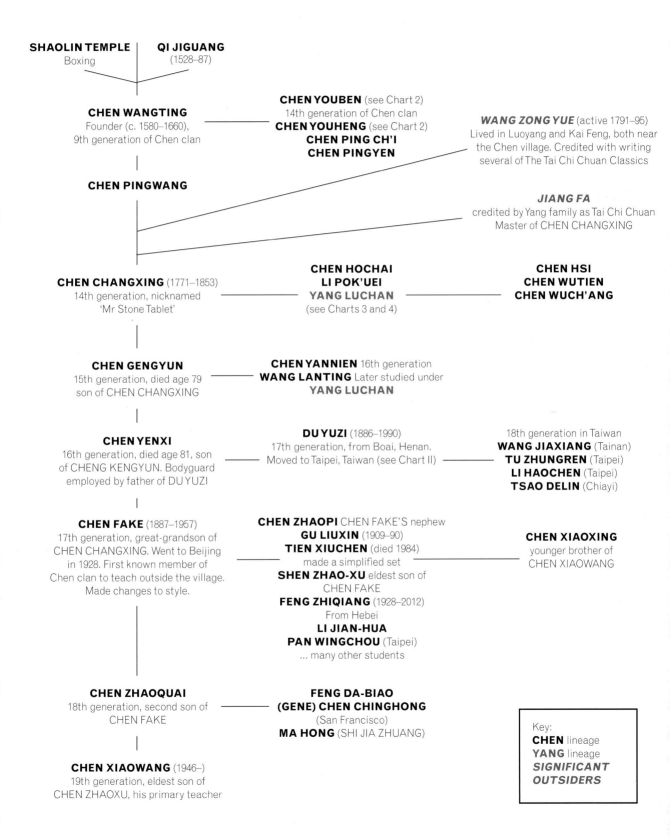

SHAOLIN TEMPLE
Boxing

QI JIGUANG
(1528–87)

CHEN WANGTING
Founder (c. 1580–1660),
9th generation of Chen clan

CHEN YOUBEN (see Chart 2)
14th generation of Chen clan
CHEN YOUHENG (see Chart 2)
CHEN PING CH'I
CHEN PINGYEN

WANG ZONG YUE (active 1791–95)
Lived in Luoyang and Kai Feng, both near
the Chen village. Credited with writing
several of The Tai Chi Chuan Classics

CHEN PINGWANG

JIANG FA
credited by Yang family as Tai Chi Chuan
Master of CHEN CHANGXING

CHEN CHANGXING (1771–1853)
14th generation, nicknamed
'Mr Stone Tablet'

CHEN HOCHAI
LI POK'UEI
YANG LUCHAN
(see Charts 3 and 4)

CHEN HSI
CHEN WUTIEN
CHEN WUCH'ANG

CHEN GENGYUN
15th generation, died age 79
son of CHEN CHANGXING

CHEN YANNIEN 16th generation
WANG LANTING Later studied under
YANG LUCHAN

CHEN YENXI
16th generation, died age 81, son
of CHENG KENGYUN. Bodyguard
employed by father of DU YUZI

DU YUZI (1886–1990)
17th generation, from Boai, Henan.
Moved to Taipei, Taiwan (see Chart II)

18th generation in Taiwan
WANG JIAXIANG (Tainan)
TU ZHUNGREN (Taipei)
LI HAOCHEN (Taipei)
TSAO DELIN (Chiayi)

CHEN FAKE (1887–1957)
17th generation, great-grandson of
CHEN CHANGXING. Went to Beijing
in 1928. First known member of
Chen clan to teach outside the village.
Made changes to style.

CHEN ZHAOPI CHEN FAKE'S nephew
GU LIUXIN (1909–90)
TIEN XIUCHEN (died 1984)
made a simplified set
SHEN ZHAO-XU eldest son of
CHEN FAKE
FENG ZHIQIANG (1928–2012)
From Hebei
LI JIAN-HUA
PAN WINGCHOU (Taipei)
... many other students

CHEN XIAOXING
younger brother of
CHEN XIAOWANG

CHEN ZHAOQUAI
18th generation, second son of
CHEN FAKE

FENG DA-BIAO
(GENE) CHEN CHINGHONG
(San Francisco)
MA HONG (SHI JIA ZHUANG)

CHEN XIAOWANG (1946–)
19th generation, eldest son of
CHEN ZHAOXU, his primary teacher

Key:
CHEN lineage
YANG lineage
SIGNIFICANT
OUTSIDERS

Chart 2: Other lineages from the Chen clan

The Twins
CHEN YOUBEN and
CHEN YOUHENG

CHEN FENG-CHANG
CHEN JISHEN (1809–65)
CHEN SANDE
CHEN BAOSHEN
CHEN TINGDUNG
CHEN ZHONGSHEN (c. 1809–71)
son of CHEN YOUBEN

CHEN SEN
CEN CHUNGLI

CHEN MIAO
CHEN T'UNG
CHEN FUYUAN
LIU CH'ANG CH'UN
CHEN XIN (1849–1929) Grand
nephew of CHEN YOUBEN
CHEN KUEI
Son of CHENZHONG-SHEN
LI JINGYEN *

CHEN QINGPING
(1795–1868) nephew of
CHEN YOUBEN.
Created Zhaobao Style.

CHANG ISHAN
CHANG KAI
HO CHAOYUAN
LI JINGYEN * First studied
under CHEN ZHONGSHEN

CHEN CHUNYUAN
(unknown–1949)
CHEN ZIMING (unknown–195
CHEN MINGBAO Nephew o
CHEN YOU BEN

DU YUZI (See CHART 1)

WU YUXIANG *and his two brothers*
(1812–80) from Yongnian country.
Combines what he learned from
YANG LUCHAN (c.1851) with the
Zhaobao Style. He learned later from
CHEN YINGPING (c. 1850) to create
Wu (Yuxiang) Style.

LI YIYU (1852–92)
Nephew of YU YUXIANG,
created his **Li Style**.

HAO WEIZHENG
(1842–1920) Created the
Hao Style.

MA TUNGWEN
LI XIANGYUAN
HAO YUERU
(1877–1935)
Son of HAO WEIZHEN

TUNG YINGJIE Learned later with
YANG CHENGFU
XU CHEN
HAO XIAOJU Grandson of
HAO WEIZHEN

SUN LUTANG
(1860–1933)
Blended Qu Style with
Xingyi and Bagua
Styles to create the
Sun Style.

SUN CHIENYUN
SUN TSUNZHOU
CHENG HUAIXIEN
From Hebei

CHANG SHIHJUNG (Taiwan)

Key:
CHEN
ZHAOBAO
WU (YU-XIANG)
LI
HAO
SUN

Chart 3: Direct Yang family lineages

YANG-LUCHAN [FUKUI] (1799–1872) Native of Yongnian Country, Hebei. Taught members of Manchu royal family and imperial guard in Beijing. Nicknamed 'YANG the Invincible' Founder of the **YANG Style**

ZHANG FENGQI
CHEN XIUFENG
LI-RUIDONG
WANG LANTING
WAN CHUN (Manchu nobles' athletic camp)
LING SHAN (Manchu nobles' athletic camp)
WU YUXIANG (1812–80) and his two brothers (see Chart 2)
QUAN YOU (see Chart 4)
YANG BANHOU (see Chart 4) (1837–92) second son of

LI PINFU
QING YI [CHING YAT] buddhist monk

QI MINXUAN

CHENG TINHUNG (author's Master)

YANG FENGHOU (1835–81) eldest son of **YANG LUCHAN**

YANG JIANHOU (1839–1917) third son of **YANG LUCHAN**, modified the form from his father

CHI DE
XU YU-SHEN (1879–1945)
YANG CHAOYUAN
YANG SHAOHOU [XIAO-HSIUNG] (1862–1929) first son of **YANG JIANHOU**

YANG CHENSHENG
TIAN SHAOXIAN

YANG CHENGFU [CHAO-QING] (1883–1936) third son of **YANG JUANHOU.** Taught in many parts of China

TUNG YONG-CHIEH (1888–1961) studied HAO Style, then with **YANG** for 20 years
FU ZHONGWEN, nephew of **YANG CHENGFU**
YANG SHOUCHUNG (Hong Kong, *1909). Eldest son of **YANG CHENGFU.**
YANG ZHENJI (Handan, Hebei), fourth son of **YANG CHENGFU**
CHEN WEIMING
LI YA-SHUAN
WU HUICHUN (unknown–1937)
CHOY HOKPENG (1886–1957), San Francisco
CHENG MANCHING (1900–57), New York

... many other students

JASMINE TUNG (Hong Kong), daughter of TUNG YINGCHIEH
TUNG FULIN (Hawaii), son of TUNG YINGCHIEH
LI HUANG CHE (Shanghai)
HUANG WEN-SHAN (Los Angeles)

IP TAI-TAK
CHU GINSOON
CHU KING HUNG (London)

LIANG CHINGYU (Hong Kong), chief disciple of CHEN WEI-MING

LIANG TUNGTSAI (*1900)
WILLIAM C.C. CHEN (New York)
CHANG CHIHKANG
HSIH SHUFENG (Taichung)
HUANG SHENGHSIEN (Singapore)

... many other students

YANG ZHEN-DUO (Taiyuan, Hebei) third son of YANG CHENGFU. (*1926). Most of his training was under his brothers, SHAUCHUNG and ZHENJI. Main representative of **YANG** family today

Key:
LI
YANG
WU
SIGNIFICANT OUTSIDERS

Chart 4: Yang and Wu lineages

**YANG-LUCHAN
[FUKUI]** (1799–1872)
Native of Yongnian
Country, Hebei. Taught
members of Manchu
royal family & imperial
guard in Beijing.
Nicknamed 'YANG the
Invincible'. Founder of the
YANG Style

YANG JIANHOU (1938–1917)
third son of **YANG LUCHAN.**
Modified the form from his father.

YANG BANHOU
(see Chart 3)
(1837–1892) second son
of **YANG LUCHAN**

CHEN XIUFENG
LING SHAN (Beijing)
WAN CH'UN
CHANG QINGLING ——— WANG YANNIEN (Taipei)
YANG CHAOP'ENG
WANG CHIAOYO (Beijing) — KUO LIENYING ——— CHIANG YUNCHUNG

QUAN YOU (1834-1902)
Manchu nobles' athletic
camp. Also studied under
YANG LUCHAN

WANG MAO-ZHAI ——— **YANG YUTING** ——— WANG PEISHENG (Beijing, *1919)
LIU FENGSHAN
QI KESAN ——————— QI MINXUAN ——— CHENG TINHUNG
*(author's master).
Started training under his uncle
CHENG WINGKWONG

WU JIANQUAN
(1970–1942) Son of
QUAN YU. Founder
of the **WU** style that
is second in popularity
to the YANG style.
This is not the same as
WU-YUXIANG's WU style

WU TZU CHEN
WANG JUNSHENG
CHU MINI, brother-in-law
of **WANG QING WEI,**
political leader
MA YUEH LIANG
(Shanghai), son-in-law of
WU JIANQUAN ——————— MA JIANGBAO (Shanghai),
son of MA YUEHLIANG

CHENG WINGKWONG — CHENG TINHUNG (1930–2005)
(author's master). Later trained
with QI MINXUAN

**WU KUNGYI
WU KUNGCHO
WU YINGHUA,**
sons & daugher of
WU JIANQUAN

Key:
YANG
WU

Bibliography

Chen Pan Ling *Original Tai Chi Chuan Textbook*
(Blitz! Design, 1998)

Cheng Man-ch'ing & Smith, Robert W *T'ai-Chi: The Supreme Ultimate Exercise for Health, Sport and Self-defence*
(Charles E. Tuttle Co., 1967)

Cheng Tin-hung *Tai Chi Transcendent Art*
(Hong Kong Tai Chi Association, 1976)

Cleary, Thomas *The Book of Balance and Harmony*
(North Point Press, 1989)

Davis, Barbara/Chen Weiming *Taiji Sword and Other Writings* (North Atlantic Books, 2002)

Davis, Barbara *The Taijiquan Classics*
(North Atlantic Books, 2004)

Docherty, Dan *Complete Tai Chi Chuan*
(The Crowood Press, 1997)

Docherty, Dan *The Tai Chi Bible*
(Godsfield Press, 2014)

Docherty, Dan *Tai Chi Chuan – Decoding the Classics for the Modern Martial Artist* (The Crowood Press, 2009)

Henricks, Robert G *Lao-Tzu: Te-Tao Ching*
(Mackays of Chatham PLC, 1990)

Jou, Tsung Hwa *The Tao of Tai-Chi Chuan*
(Tai Chi Foundation, 1981)

Lao, Tzu *Tao Te Ching* (Penguin Books, 1963)

Legge, James *The Texts of Taoism: The Tao Te Ching of Lao Tzu, The Writings of Chuang Tzu*
(Dover Publications, 1962)

Needham, Joseph *Science and Civilisation in China*
(Cambridge University Press, 1983)

Palmer, David A *Qigong Fever*
(C. Hurst & Co., 2007)

Paludan, Ann *Chronicle of the Chinese Emperors: The Reign-By-Reign Record of the Rulers of Imperial China*
(Thames and Hudson, 1998)

Ronan, Colin A *The Shorter Science and Civilisation in China* (Cambridge University Press, 1978)

Roth, Harold D *Original Tao – Inward Training and the Foundations of Taoist Mysticism*
(Columbia University Press, 1999)

Sawyer, Ralph D *The Seven Military Classics of Ancient China* (Westview Press,1993)

Smith, Robert W *Chinese Boxing: Masters and Methods*
(North Atlantic Books, 1974)

Wang Peisheng/Zeng Weiqi *Wu Style Taijiquan*
(Hai Feng Publishing Co.,1983)

Wayne, Peter M *Harvard Medical School Guide to Tai Chi: 12 Weeks to a Healthy Body, Strong Heart and Sharp Mind* (Shambhala Publications, 2013)

Wells, Marnix *The Pheasant Cap Master and the End of History* (Three Pines Press, 2013)

Wells, Marnix *Scholar Boxer: Chang Naizhou's Theory of Internal Martial Arts and the Evolution of Taijiquan* (North Atlantic Books, 2005)

Werner, ETC *Myths and Legends of China*
(Graham Brash Ltd, 1984)

Wile, Douglas *Lost Tai Chi Classics from the Late Ching Dynasty* (State University of New York Press, 1996)

Wile, Douglas *Tai Chi Ancestors* (Sweet ch'i Press, 1999.)

Wile, Douglas *T'ai-chi Touchstones: Yang Family Secret Transmissions* (Sweet Ch'i Press, 1983)

Williams, CAS *Outlines of Chinese Symbolism and Art Motives* (Dover Publications, 1976)

Wong, Hon Shiu *Investigations into the Authenticity of the Chang San-Feng Ch'uan-Chi: The Complete Works of Chang San-Feng* (The Australian National University Press, 1982)

Wu, K.C. *Wu Style Tai Chi Chuan* (Jonathan Krehm on behalf of Wu Style Tai Chi Chuan Federation, 2006)

Yang, Jwing-Ming. *Tai Chi Secrets of the Wu Style*
(YMAA Publication Center, 2002)

Yang, Zhendou *Yang style Taijiquan*
(Hai Feng Publishing House, 1988)

The Yellow Emperor's Canon of Internal Medicine
(China Science & Technology Press, 1997)

Index

Index cont.

Picture Credits

Main photography: Octopus Publishing Group/
Ruth Jenkinson.

Other photography:
Alamy Ivy Close Images 41 below.
Bridgeman Images Indianapolis Museum of Art, USA/
  Mr and Mrs Richard Crane Fund 34; Societe Asiatique,
  College de France, Paris, France/Archives Charmet 14.
Corbis 13/Dougal Waters/Digital Vision/Ocean 226; Chen
  Haining/Xinhua Press 57.
David Durrant 214, 215, 216, 217, 219.
Getty Images Herve BRUHAT/Gamma-Rapho 51;
  Howard Sochurek/The LIFE Picture Collection 37;
  Karl Johaentges 45; Popperfoto 36; TAO Images
  Limited 33; View Stock 39.
James Connachan 87.
Photoshot Xu Hongxing/Xinhua 67, 201, 224–225.
Shutterstock Eva Ziskova 15; Kim Briers 54–55.
SuperStock Iberfoto/Iberfoto 35.
TopFoto The Granger Collection 24 right.
Tatiana Kramtsova 203.
via Wikipedia Gisling 56.
Wellcome Library, London 82-83.

Author's Acknowledgements

In researching *The Complete Tai Chi Tutor*, I've come to
see that I've long harboured many unknown knowns
(things I thought I knew, but which I really didn't)
regarding all aspects of the art, especially its purity.
On my Tai Chi road to Damascus many good folk helped
and guided me. Thanks to Dr. Alex Ryan for her help
on the structure of this book; to Birgit Muller from the
University of Aachen for her work on maps, charts and
diagrams, and to my Chinese teacher, Moira Ni, for the
great calligraphy.

Many thanks also to Paju Becker from Finland and
Emma Åkesson from Sweden, the two stars of the book,
and to the excellent supporting cast of Cuong Sam,
Alan Austin, Charles Glasser, Kevin White, Alina Kisina,
Ainara Becker and Ronan Docherty.

Finally thanks to my editors, Liz and Sybella.

Credits

Executive Editor: Liz Dean
Managing Editor: Sybella Stephens
Deputy Art Director: Yasia Williams-Leedham
Designer: Geoff Borin
Photographer: Ruth Jenkinson
Picture Researcher: Jennifer Veall
Models: Emma Åkesson, Alan Austin, Paju Becker,
  Ainara Becker, Ronan Docherty, Charles Glasser,
  Alina Kisina, Cuong Sam, Kevin White
Hair & Make up: Roisin Donaghy, Victoria Barnes
Production Controller: Allison Gonsalves